TRADITIONAL CHINESE MEDICINE

A GUIDE TO ITS PRACTICE

D1826664

TRADITIONAL CHINESE MEDICINE

A GUIDE TO ITS PRACTICE

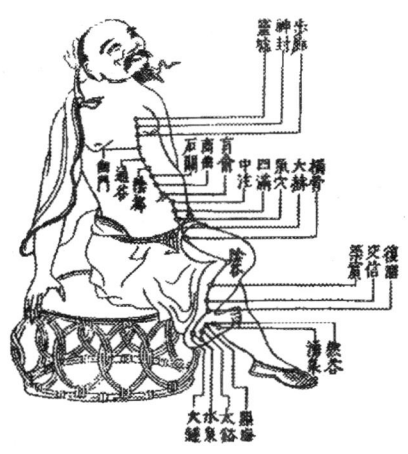

REY TIQUIA

A**CHOICE**BOOK

This book is dedicated to my wife
Margaret Roslyn Fuary
and my daughter
Ana-Marikit Tiquia

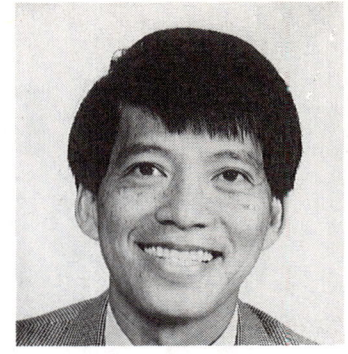

TRADITIONAL CHINESE MEDICINE

First published in 1996 by CHOICE Books, a division of the Australian
Consumers' Association, 57 Carrington Road, Marrickville NSW 2204

National Library of Australia
Cataloguing-in-publication data:

Tiquia, Rey.
Traditional Chinese medicine: a guide to its practice.

Bibliography.
Includes index.
ISBN 0 947277 20 X

1. Medicine, Chinese. 2. Medicine, Chinese - Australia.
I. Title.

610.951

Printed in Australia by Australian Print Group
Typeset by All Language Typesetters
Designed by Jack Jagtenberg
Edited by Louise Egerton

CONTENTS

FOREWORD

There have been many attempts to present the complex body of knowledge known generally as traditional Chinese medicine in terms that Westerners can readily understand. Part of the problem faced by any presenter is the vast complexity of that body of knowledge. Developing in China across millennia, absorbing and modifying multiple cultural influences, traditional Chinese medicine, like Western scientific medicine, is far from a coherent and unified body of knowledge. It is rich in contrast and heterogeneity; and that is precisely its strength in the modern world.

This book is unusual because its unifying theme is a focus on practices of traditional Chinese medicine. It offers a clear way of seeing how the practices of diagnosis in traditional Chinese medicine are linked to the practices of treatment. Showing this link, and how it differs from Western scientific medicine is achieved through offering a clear account of 'the big picture' of traditional Chinese medicine.

We don't usually talk about 'big pictures'; we take them for granted. And that 'taking for granted' can cause problems. Let's look briefly at the 'big picture' of the practice of Western scientific medicine as a way of sensitising ourselves to some of what we normally take for granted in the practice of medicine. The stories that we as patients go away with, after a visit to a Western doctor, usually relate to some entity that is present but should not be present — a flu virus in cells, or fatty deposits in the blood vessels of our heart. Or the story might relate to the absence of an entity — not enough pressure in the blood vessels; not enough glucose in the blood. It's a mapping story. Western doctors map the presences and absences of a vast range of things in our unwell bodies. And they have a vast technology to help in this mapping enterprise. This mapping is seen as a first step in working towards putting the machine of the body back into good working order.

The stories that we go away with after a visit to a practitioner of traditional Chinese medicine are very different. And that is the reason we need a book like this one. This book alerts us to the 'stories behind' the practice of traditional Chinese medicine, and how they relate to what it is that doctors of traditional Chinese medicine do. It helps us begin to learn how to be patients of a doctor of traditional Chinese medicine.

Rey Tiquia's book helps us to understand that traditional Chinese medicine is not about getting a map of what's present and what's absent in the body; its about picturing balance and harmony. And there are different ways of picturing balance. We see that the 'story behind' traditional Chinese medicine is actually a composite picture; a working together of varying ways of picturing balance. Working different ways of picturing balance together can give a precise and sensitive way to detect and represent imbalance, and provide a framework for recommendations to restore balance.

"Yin and Yang", "the Five Elements" and "Qi" are the names given to the three main ways of picturing balance which have been 'massaged' together over centuries of practice of traditional Chinese medicine, to give a working matrix for detecting imbalance. These are the elements of the stories we take away with us when we are patients of doctors of traditional Chinese medicine. Rey Tiquia literally helps us come to terms with these ways of picturing balance. He gives us the words.

The differences between traditional Chinese medicine and Western scientific medicine in the ways they picture health and illness mean of course that the practices of diagnosis, and the practices of treatment in the two traditions are different. But they also mean that the experience of, and the practices associated with being a patient of a doctor of traditional Chinese medicine are quite different to being the patient of a Western doctor.

Practices of being a patient? Surely a patient just has to be ill. But is it as simple as this? If you think about it you'll soon see that when we visit a Western medical practitioner we feel we need to have our story straight. We put some time into rehearsing our story of our pains and discomforts. Very often we will even identify that there are particular things that we feel are present in or absent from our bodies.

In Australia for the most part we have learned to be the patients of doctors practising a particular brand of scientific Western medicine. But as more and more of us realise the benefits of traditional Chinese medicine we need to learn how to be effective patients in this system of health care. We need to learn to understand ourselves within the 'stories' of this rich tradition of knowing. And it is in this endeavour that Rey Tiquia's book is particularly helpful.

Dr Helen Verran
Department of History and Philosophy of Science
University of Melbourne

PREFACE 前言

The main purpose of this book is to promote awareness of Traditional Chinese Medicine (TCM). As TCM continues to develop in China and internationally, people increasingly ask for precise information about this knowledge system. Questions commonly raised are: What is traditional Chinese medicine? What are its origins? How is it done? What are its disciplines? Does it work?

At present, most of the available literature on this subject is in the Chinese language, with English-language materials being limited to specific topics and generally catering for students or practitioners of TCM. Most books deal separately with the various disciplines, i.e. acupuncture, herbal medicine, food therapy, tuina massage and nurturing life. Most, too, are highly theoretical and generally vague about the TCM system of diagnosis.

This book is unparalleled, both in and out of China, in that it presents TCM in a manner that has never been presented before. It opens by describing, clearly and practically, the framework of TCM practice: how it is done and its mechanism of diagnosis. It goes on to explain the unique concept of clinical patterns in TCM diagnosis and how they are linked with the principles for tailoring individual treatment. This system of diagnosis is then put into the context of TCM's main therapeutic disciplines of herbal medicine, acupuncture, food therapy, tuina and nurturing life, each of which is dealt with in considerable detail.

In weaving together the various elements of TCM practice, the bulk of the reference material referred to when writing this book came from classical and contemporary Chinese language sources. Some, too, came from contemporary Chinese literature that mixes TCM and biomedical concepts in what is often a decontextualised, hence confusing, manner. Identifying the essential aspects of TCM practice amidst all these volumes and transforming them into a meaningful and easily understood work has been the greatest challenge in writing this book. Hopefully, the product is a unique focus on the practice of TCM.

The author has been working for a number of years on how best to present some of the subtle concepts and ideas of TCM. His practice and his current postgraduate studies at Melbourne University on 'Developing Criteria for the Standards Practice of TCM in Australia' has been the impetus for the informative approach of this book. Many lectures and articles in mainstream newspapers, magazines and journals in Australia have been refocused, expanded and integrated into the work. The intention has been to write a well-rounded, practical and clearly understood book for everyone interested in learning more about the TCM body of knowledge.

Rey Tiquia

AKNOWLEDGEMENTS

I am very grateful to three individuals who contributed enormously, either directly or indirectly, in the writing of this book. First of all, I would like to thank my wife, Margaret Roslyn Fuary, a teacher of Mandarin, for initially editing and proofreading this manuscript. I am eternally grateful for the constant guidance and support she has provided in my efforts to make TCM come to life in a Western environment.

Second, I would like to express my gratitude to my mentor and teacher, Dr Helen Watson-Verran, the Director of the 'Science in Society Program' at the Department of History and Philosophy of Science, Melbourne University, for her valuable philosophical direction and guidance which greatly influenced the main philosophical thrust of this book. In a sense, this book is inspired by the wonderful work that Helen is doing in the area of cross-cultural communication.

Third, I would like to thank Mr Steven Clavey for his helpful and constructive comments.

I am grateful to all of my patients, who, with their trust and confidence, have made my fruitful TCM practice in Australia possible. Each and everyone of them are essential contributors in the weaving of this book.

Finally, I wish to pay homage to my TCM mentors in China, specifically, those from my alma mater, the Beijing College of TCM. Their unselfish devotion to the practice of TCM 'in the service of the people' will always inspire me in my endeavours.

Rey Tiquia

THE PRACTICE OF TRADITIONAL CHINESE MEDICINE (TCM)

IN DEFINING TRADITIONAL CHINESE MEDICINE (TCM), WE SHOULD INITIALLY examine the two original Chinese characters which refer to it, i.e. 'zhong' 中 and 'yi' 醫.

According to Confucian doctrine, 'zhong' means centre, halfway between two extremes or the mean. 'Zhong' also means China or Chinese and today this is its primary meaning. 'Yi' means medicine, to cure or a doctor. So 'zhong yi' is the term commonly used for Chinese medicine, as opposed to 'xi yi', which means Western medicine. Prior to the advent of Western medicine, Chinese medicine was simply known as 'yi'.

The three components of the ideographic script for the word 'yi' indicate the essence of TCM practice. The upper left portion of the script is made up of an arrowhead 矢 in a quiver ⌐. The right side portion is a picture of a right hand 又 about to strike. Together this means targeting the arrow against the evil influences that cause disease. The upper component of the script 殳 then refers to Chinese medicine's method of diagnosing a condition, i.e. accurately pinpointing a disease pattern. The lower portion 酉 represents an ancient vase used for storing fermented liquor. This is also the vessel in which medicinal decoctions or elixirs were prepared and taken.

Thus, from its ideographic meaning, TCM or 'zhong yi' refers to a system of medicine which puts a premium on balance and moderation and uses herbal decoctions to specifically and accurately target a disease pattern.

DEFINING THE PRACTICE OF TCM

In further defining TCM we must examine how it is done and how it works, i.e. its practice.

TCM is a body of medical knowledge that has emerged, developed and been systematised over a period of four thousand years. Chinese social, philosophical and cultural practice has provided the contextual background for its development and it is even today the Chinese people's principal practice of maintaining health and fighting off diseases.

The practices of TCM form a coherent body of knowledge which includes a unique method of recognising disease phenomena. It encompasses a variety of therapeutic methods, such as herbal and food therapy, acupuncture and tuina (massage), and includes a range of disease-preventative methods like Qi Gong, Tai Ji Quan and Yang Sheng or 'nurturing life'. (These terms are explained later.)

Whilst the practice of TCM is clearly defined in the Chinese context, in the West an undue focus has been given to theoretical definitions of TCM, isolating it from its contextual background. As a result, many aspects of TCM's practice have been cannibalised and mechanically integrated with other knowledge systems. A graphic illustration of this is acupuncture, which is one of the cornerstone practices of the TCM body of knowledge.

Decontextualised or mechanically detached from its life context, we find several acupuncture hybrids, e.g. 'medical acupuncture', 'meridian acupuncture', 'Chakra acupuncture' and even 'naturopathic acupuncture'.

While the appropriation of certain aspects of the TCM body of knowledge is inevitable, there is a clear need for it to be done with greater understanding and sensitivity. Uprooting 'bits' of TCM theories out of their historical, social and cultural context and then mechanically combining these with 'bits' of other medical knowledge systems can only lead to an unhealthy cross-fertilisation and confusion. Hence, there is a need to move away from this purely theoretical approach to understanding TCM. The best way to understand and explain TCM is to present it in terms of how it is done and how it works. This is the aim of this book.

THE CONTENT OF TCM PRACTICE

The practice of TCM can be summed up in four Chinese words: 'bian zheng lun zhi' 辨证论治. This translates as 'proposing treatment principles in accordance with the clinical pattern'. 'Bian' means to differentiate; 'zheng' means evidence of clinical patterns; 'lun' means in accordance with; while 'zhi' means treatment.

From this translation it is apparent that the practice of TCM involves two aspects. One is the investigative and diagnostic phase of differentiating clinical patterns which in Chinese is referred to as 'bian zheng'.

The second phase is the practical tailoring and administration of appropriate treatment to a patient, which in Chinese is called 'lun zhi'. In TCM, the treatment administered (lun zhi) depends upon the presenting clinical patterns or 'zheng'.

DIFFERENTIATING CLINICAL PATTERNS — A BASIS FOR DIAGNOSIS

What are clinical patterns in TCM? How do they become the basis of diagnosis in TCM?

The concept of clinical patterns is a process that is unique to TCM. It is the core of the investigative, cognitive and diagnostic process of doing TCM. People often confuse this process with the orthodox Western medicine's concept of disease syndromes or diseases' symptoms and signs.

In TCM, a person who is healthy manifests signs of health, balance and harmony. A healthy pulse beats five times per breath, and all the corresponding regions of the pulse beat at an even and consistent rate, rhythm, strength, manifesting a specific pattern. The tongue is pinkish in colour with a thin white coat and normal texture. Most importantly, a healthy person is free from any discomfort or pain, has a vigorous spirit, robust physical build and leads a balanced life which includes a good appetite, a regular sleeping pattern and a reasonable amount of exercise. Signs or symptoms which are at variance with the above emerge as patterns of disease, clinical patterns or 'zheng hou'.

'Zheng hou' 证候 is the complete Chinese name for the concept of 'clinical patterns'. 'Zheng' by itself means evidence of, proof, to prove, to demonstrate; while 'hou' means a condition which is in a state of flux, to keep watch, to detect, to survey, or to examine.

The Chinese script for 'hou' 候 like that for 'yi' (medicine) also has a script component 矢 representing an arrowhead. The whole Chinese script represents an arrow fixed on a target. 'Zheng hou' together then means evidence of a condition which is in a state of flux and detected under close examination.

In TCM, diseases or 'ji bing' 疾病 are seen as human pain and suffering. Clinical patterns are signs and symptoms which emerge at a specific stage in the overall development of a disease. They are reactions to disease-causing factors. The specific clinical pattern determines the specific therapeutic approach or management.

To establish the clinical pattern of a disease the practitioner goes through two investigative and cognitive stages. The first stage involves the use of the 'Four Examination Techniques' of looking, listening and smelling, inquiring, and palpating. This stage involves collecting data from the presenting signs and symptoms of a patient. The subsequent stage involves the analysis, synthesis and verification of the data collected. This phase draws upon TCM 'conceptual templates'. In order to fully understand some of the terms that follow it is essential to familiarise yourself with the explanations on pages 33 to 37. An understanding of Qi will be helpful too, and can be attained from page 35 in Chapter 2.

STAGE ONE: THE FOUR EXAMINATION TECHNIQUES *Si Zhen* 四诊

1. Observing *WANG ZHEN* 望诊

Looking at and observing the patient is one of the most important examination techniques used to establish a clinical pattern. In order to understand the inner dynamics of the body, a practitioner looks for signs and symptoms reflected in the outer body shell. These external manifestations are like 'shadows' of the workings of the internal organs.

Examining the patient's signs and symptoms establishes the visual contours of a clinical pattern. The practitioner collects data on the patient's spirit, facial colour, physical build and the colour and structure of the tongue.

Spirit *Shen* 神

The spirit here corresponds to the external spiritual manifestations of a patient's physical being. It is the concentrated manifestation of life activities, and includes consciousness, the thinking process and emotional dispositions. In TCM, the eyes best reflect the state of the spirit.

Alert and sparkling eyes, a clear mind, clear coherent speech and normal reflexes constitute the patterns of a person who 'has a good spirit' (de shen). A patient with such a spirit has strong anti-pathogenic Qi (zheng Qi) which means recovery from an illness will be strong. (See glossary for an explanation of anti-pathogenic Qi.)

On the other hand, when the eyes have an indifferent look, are dull, and slow in responding, this indicates that the patient 'has lost the spirit' (shi shen). This particular clinical pattern shows that the anti-pathogenic Qi is weak, thereby making it possible for deterioration even in the case of a slight illness.

Facial Colours *Se* 色

Observing the facial colour may be compared with looking at the sky to detect weather changes. Facial colour can indicate illness. For Chinese, Koreans, Vietnamese and Japanese, the normal facial colour is a slightly lustrous, yellowish pinkish complexion. For Europeans, it would be a slightly lustrous pinkish white complexion, and for those with brown or black facial colour, such as Africans, Polynesians, etc., the complexion should also be slightly lustrous. Complexions tinged with shades of green, white, red, black or yellow may indicate illness.

In general, a pale or white complexion may indicate a blood or Qi deficiency (which is similar to symptoms of anaemia), while a reddish facial complexion may indicate a hot clinical pattern. A greenish or bluish facial complexion may indicate a cold clinical pattern, while a yellow facial colour may indicate a deficient or damp clinical pattern.

Physical Build *Xing* 形

This aspect of looking into a patient's condition focuses on their overall physical build. A strong and healthy physical build reflects strong and healthy inner organ systems.

In general terms, physical build is the reflection of the body's blood vessels running near the surface and its tendons, skin and bone structures. In TCM theory, these tissues or organs are extensions of inner organ systems. The tendons are an extension of the liver system; the blood vessels, an extension of the heart system; the skin, an extension of the lung system; and the bones are extensions of the kidney system. Abnormal manifestations of any of these external tissues or organs are barometers of the workings of the inner organ systems.

In addition, an examination is made of a patient's overall physical constitution. Such features as weight, muscle and tendon growth, bone and skin condition and any abnormal outgrowth on the surface of the body are noted.

Looking at the tongue *Bian She* 辨舌

Looking at the tongue is one of the most important examination techniques in TCM. There is an ancient Chinese saying which goes, 'the tongue is the mirror of the inner organ systems'. This means that by examining changes of the tongue, one can detect changes in the disease condition of the internal organ systems.

To examine the tongue properly, one must expose the tongue to natural sunlight. When seeing a TCM practitioner, show the tongue in a relaxed and natural manner. Poke out as much of the tongue (which should include the back region of the tongue) as one can without overstraining the tongue muscles. Spread the tongue as it poked out before examination. Avoid taking any food with food colours, e.g. strawberry lollies, coloured chewing gums or drinks, as these foods can affect the tongue's natural colour and coating.

Features to be noted include the tongue's coating, the tongue proper (the muscular tissues and the external contours of the blood vessels), the tongue's colour, its movement and moisture. Tongue coating can indicate how severely a pathogenic Qi (disease-causing agent) has affected the body, while the state of the muscular tissue and blood vessels can indicate imbalances (deficiencies or excesses) among the internal organ systems. A normal healthy tongue with 'spirit' is pinkish, pale red in colour, moist, moves freely and has a thin white moist coating.

A red-coloured tongue is an indication of an abnormal condition. This is an indication of a hot clinical pattern due to invasion by external wind-heat pathogenic Qi, a clinical phenomenon common to those with high fever due to viral infections.

A red tongue proper may also indicate a deficient clinical pattern of a particular organ system generated from within an inner organ system, e.g. the kidney organ system (see pages 36 to 37). This is similar to conditions of unexplained low-grade fever among some patients with chronic diseases.

Another example of an abnormal tongue condition is a 'flabby tongue', which may be described as being broader and bigger than a normal tongue.

A flabby tongue may be an indication of dampness or mucus build-up due to spleen system deficiency.

An ulcerated, cracked tongue or thorny tongue is also an abnormal condition. (A thorny tongue has projections on most of its surface.)

Some abnormal tongue coatings are yellow, grey or white. A yellow coating may be further differentiated into thin, thick, sticky or dry. A thin yellow coating indicates an external hot clinical pattern; a thick yellow coat indicates an excess of a hot clinical pattern of the stomach system; a yellow sticky coating indicates accumulation of damp heat in the interior; while a dry yellow coat indicates an excess hot clinical pattern of the stomach and intestines systems due to deficiency in body fluids.

Data derived from examination of the tongue is combined with other presenting symptoms and signs to establish and diagnose a clinical pattern.

2. Listening and Smelling WEN ZHEN 闻诊

Listening to body sounds and smelling body odours are important sources of data when establishing clinical patterns. While looking can establish the 'shadows' of the internal organs' workings, body sounds can be compared with their 'echoes' and body odours, their 'scent'.

Body sounds include the patient's speech, breathing and pathological sounds, e.g. coughing. Certain sounds have been correlated with the functioning of certain organ systems. For example, shouting is associated with the liver system; weeping with the lung system; singing musical sounds with the spleen system; moaning and groaning with the kidney system; and laughter with the heart system. Sneezing, hiccups, stuttering, abdominal sounds, etc. are also some of the body sounds that should be taken into consideration when establishing the clinical pattern. Listening closely to these sounds can lead to an understanding of how well these organ systems are functioning.

Body smells refer to body scents emanating from the surface of the body. A healthy person whose Qi and blood are flowing freely should not have any distinctive body smell or odour. However, when the Qi and blood do not circulate freely due to certain pathological factors, abnormal odours will occur. These may be manifested in the breath, perspiration, nasal discharge, in sputum, stools, urine, menstrual or vaginal discharge.

Normal breathing should be gentle, placid and even. When external pathogenic factors affect the lungs, breathing can become coarse and rapid. When the anti-pathogenic Qi of the body has been weakened then breathing can become faint, weak and slow. Coarse breathing, wheezing or a rattling sound in the chest indicate a clinical pattern whereby phlegm and heat are affecting the lung system.

In general terms, a stench similar to that of a rotten fish indicates an excessively hot clinical pattern; an acidic smell in the mouth indicates heat in the stomach or intestines; and an acidic smell in stools indicates heat in the intestines. A urine stench can indicate a pattern of damp heat in the urinary bladder system, while an exceptionally smelly 'wind' indicates heat or food stagnation in the abdomen.

With the proliferation of the use of various types of perfume, fragrant soaps, body lotions etc., real body odours are now easily concealed from the investigation of a TCM practitioner. Hence, when seeing a TCM doctor, it is best to avoid the use of perfume and other artificial beauty aids. This will greatly help the practitioner to establish the clinical pattern accurately.

3. Inquiry WEN ZHEN 问诊

Inquiry or 'Wen zhen' means examination by asking some questions. The object of the inquiry is to understand the onset and development of the illness, the response to therapy and the patient's subjective complaints. The inquiry is directed either to the patient or the patient's close relatives or friends. The aim of the inquiry is to gather data that is inaccessible through the other three methods of examination, i.e. looking, listening and smelling, and palpation. Asking relevant questions can also confirm the veracity of data already gathered.

The scope of the inquiry includes the current signs and symptoms, the history of the condition and the patient's lifestyle. Utmost trust between the practitioner and the patient is vital in the conduct of TCM inquiry. The correct congenial atmosphere must be established by the practitioner to enable the patient to voluntarily provide information about his or her illness. In addition, the inquiry should be conducted in an orderly fashion, planned in stages and focused upon certain points vital to the establishment of a clinical pattern.

The 'Ten questions verse'

The 'ten questions verse' is a rhyming poem composed by a medical scholar by the name of Zhang Jing Yue in the Ming Dynasty (AD 1368–1644). The poem lists ten items which should be considered when inquiring about the signs and symptoms of the patient. They are: chills and fevers, perspiration, pain, stool and urine, food and drinks, sleep, menstruation, history of signs and symptoms, lifestyle, and presenting signs and symptoms.

Chills and Fevers *Han Re* 寒热

Chills and fever refer to the patient's subjective feeling of either being feverish or feeling a chill. The degree to which a patient feels either of these symptoms may be used as a way of determining whether a clinical pattern is exterior or interior; yin or yang, excessive or deficient.

Fever combined with an aversion to cold occuring at the beginning of an illness indicates invasion of the body by external pathogenic Qi. If aversion to cold is the dominant symptom, then the clinical pattern may be that of external wind-cold pattern. However, if fever is the dominant symptom, then it is an external wind-heat pattern. Inquiry about chills and fever is very commonly used for upper respiratory tract or acute infections. Knowledge about chills or fevers can sometimes be crucial in establishing an accurate clinical pattern.

Perspiration or Sweating *Han* 汗

According to the theory of TCM, abnormal patterns of sweating are brought about by disharmony in the circulation of the Qi at the surface of the body. Knowledge of the degree, time and frequency of sweating can give some idea of the condition of the body's Qi.

Night sweats are a sign of deficiency of the yin, and excess of the yang Qi of the body. Frequent spontaneous sweating which may be brought on by slight physical exertion is caused by yang Qi deficiency. Profuse sweating in cases of severe illnesses is a critical sign that the yang Qi is about to be completely exhausted.

Pain *Tong* 痛

'Tong' 痛 is the Chinese word and character for pain. This Chinese script is made up of two components. The outer part refers generally to all illness. It is a symbol which can be interpreted as a sick person leaning against something. The inner character 甬 means a paved path leading to a main hall or to a tomb.

'Tong' means ache or pain; or going to extremes or sorrow. A Chinese medical scholar by the name of Li Dong Yuan, who lived during the time of the Jin Yuan dynasty in China (AD 1115–138), put forward the theory that pain is brought about by blockage or obstruction in the acupuncture channel system. Pain or 'tong' may be classified as deficient or excessive, yin or yang, hot or cold, internal or external according to its location, nature, features and duration.

Pain that is aggravated by pressure or palpation is an excessive type of pain which may result from invasion by external pathogenic Qi, obstruction of the acupuncture channels, obstruction by phlegm or food retention.

On the other hand, pain relieved by pressure or palpation is a deficient type of pain which is caused by blood or Qi deficiency along the acupuncture channels. This clinical pattern can be observed among patients with stomach or duodenal ulcers who often suffer lingering abdominal pains.

Pain that is relieved by warmth (hot or warm packs) is considered to be pain of the cold type, while pain relieved by cold or ice packs is that of the hot type. Migrating pain is caused by wind external pathogenic Qi affecting the acupuncture channels, while pain which stays in just one spot is due to obstruction of acupuncture channels by cold or damp pathogenic factors or Qi stagnation.

Pain above the diaphragm usually indicates disorders affecting the heart or lung systems; pain in the epigastric region indicates disorders affecting the spleen and stomach systems; pain below the umbilicus and in the lower abdomen indicates disorders affecting the kidney, urinary bladder or large intestine systems.

Stool and Urine *Er Bian* 二便

Inquiring about stool and urine is one of the TCM examinations which requires tact and sensitivity. Questions asked relate to colour, smell, frequency, form, texture or pain. Answers to these queries will help in determining the patient's overall clinical pattern.

A dry stool among patients who may be constipated, for example, is attributed to heat in the large intestine system which may be of an excessive type. A dry stool and constipation in patients who have had a protracted illness or after childbirth, however, is a manifestation of a deficient clinical pattern.

Diarrhoea or loose bowel motions with undigested food indicates a deficiency of the yang Qi in the spleen and stomach systems.

Yellow coloured urine shows heat of the excessive type, while clear urine in large quantities indicates a cold pattern of a deficiency type.

Food and Drink *Yin Shi* 饮食

Inquiring about what a patient eats and drinks gives a practitioner an indication of how a patient's digestive system functions as well as the condition of other internal organ systems. Patients who prefer to eat cold food and beverages may display a hot clinical pattern, while those who prefer hot food and beverages show a cold clinical pattern. A poor appetite, absence of taste in the mouth and fullness in the epigastrium can indicate a deficient spleen and stomach system. Foul belching, acid regurgitation and disgust at the sight of food after too much intake indicates food retention. Severe thirst with a desire to take fluids is an indication of an internal heat clinical pattern, while thirst without any desire to take in fluid is a indication of a pathogen cold damp invasion.

Sleep *Shui Mian* 睡眠

Inquiry into this aspect focuses on the patient's pattern of sleep, i.e. duration, disruptions, ease of sleep, dreams and nightmares. Two most common sleeping disorders are insomnia and 'addiction to sleep'.

Menstruation *Yue Jing* 月经

Women patients should always be asked about menstruation. The inquiry normally focuses on frequency, duration, amount and colour of menstrual discharge. The number of pads or tampons used can sometimes indicate quantity of discharge. This aspect of the examination is usually conducted in a gentle considerate manner.

History of signs and symptoms *Bing Shi* 病史

This is an inquiry about the course of a disease as well as its signs and symptoms. Emphasis is on correlating the occurrence of the disease with climatic conditions, lifestyle and habits, as well as injury or trauma.

Lifestyle *Sheng Huo Xi·Guan* 生活习惯
This inquiry is about eating and sleeping habits, addictions, workplace activities and daily routine. In some cases inquiring about lifestyle can reveal certain weak links in the health of a patient which need to be remedied to restore balance.

Presenting signs and symptoms *Xian Zheng Zhuang* 现症状
Presenting signs and symptoms are the main target in establishing the clinical pattern. Data established in the course of the Four Examination Techniques are correlated with the presenting signs and symptoms and then verified through inquiry.

4. Palpation QIE ZHEN 切诊
Palpation, or 'qie zhen' in Chinese, is a method of examination involving the use of the fingers or hand to feel, touch or press segments of the body surface to ascertain changes in the condition of the body. There are two major techniques of palpation used in TCM, one is feeling the pulse or 'pulse examination' and the other is palpation of various regions of the body surface like the chest, the back, the limbs, and acupuncture points and acupuncture channels.

Pulse Examination *Mai Zhen* 脉诊
Pulse examination involves the use of the three fingertips to feel both the left and right wrist pulses of the patient. These are known as the radial pulses and they are seen in TCM as a microcosm of the body's internal organ systems.

The pulses are divided into three equal regions or segments: the 'inch', 'bar' and 'foot' ('cun', 'guan' and 'chi' in Chinese). The segment closest to the wrist is the inch; it corresponds to internal organ systems on the upper part of the body, i.e. the heart and lung systems. That segment in the middle is the bar; it corresponds to organ systems in the middle segment of the body, i.e. the spleen, stomach, liver and gall bladder systems. The final segment farthest from the

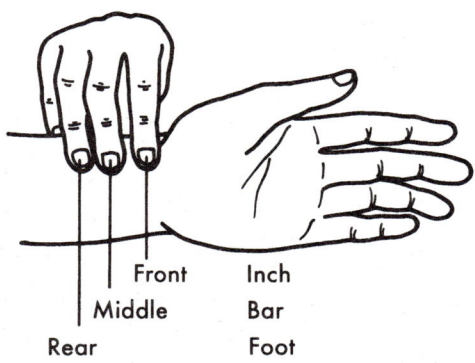

Front   Inch
Middle   Bar
Rear   Foot

Pulse Positions

wrist is the foot. This segment corresponds to the organ systems in the lower section of the body, i.e. the kidney and urinary bladder systems.

The pulse is also segmented vertically into what is referred to as the 'nine states of condition' (jiu hou). Combining the horizontal and vertical methods of feeling the radial pulse of both hands allows the practitioner to understand the conditions of internal organ systems from a different perspective.

When examining the pulse, the practitioner must be relaxed, attentive and free from distractions. The patient, too, should be relaxed and must not have been through any recent strenuous activity and or stressful situation. The best time to take the pulse is early in the morning. However, the pulse may also be felt at other times of the day.

Each wrist is lain upon a small pulse pillow. The wrist must be level with the table or ground. This ensures a normal flow of blood along the radial pulse. First, the practitioner feels the entire contour of the radial pulse of both hands. Then the nature and configuration of each segment of the pulse is examined. The practitioner first places the tip of his or her middle finger upon the bar segment of the pulse, then the index and ring fingers follow upon the inch and foot segments respectively.

By applying graduations of pressure — light, medium and heavy — on these segments, the frequency (or rate), rhythm, length, strength, shape, size, quality and specific pattern of the pulse is monitored. Abnormal changes in any segment can be ascertained by exerting an even pressure on all three regions of the pulse, then feeling the configuration of each segment and comparing one with another. Below is a table of pulse segments and the areas of the body to which they pertain.

Left hand	inch	light pressure	small intestines
		heavy pressure	heart
	bar	light pressure	gall bladder
		heavy pressure	liver
	foot	light pressure	urinary bladder
		heavy pressure	kidneys
Right hand	inch	light pressure	large intestines
		heavy pressure	lungs
	bar	light pressure	stomach
		heavy pressure	spleen
	foot	light pressure	kidney
		heavy pressure	gate of life

The Normal Pulse

A normal pulse has a rate or frequency of 4–5 beats per breath. It must have a regular rhythm and an even beat. It must not be too superficial, short, wide, narrow, thin, strong or weak. It should be felt upon placing the fingers over it.

All pulse regions and their vertical depths representing internal organ systems in the body also have their respective normal parameters.

For example, the pulse corresponding to the heart organ system ('inch' region of the left radial pulse where heavy finger pressure is applied) normally should be round and smooth like 'the beads of pearls flowing smoothly'. The pulse corresponding to the lung organ system ('inch' region of the right radial pulse where heavy finger pressure is applied) is normally neither too fast nor slow, but light and soft to touch, and flows with ease like the 'pod from the elm tree being blown down by the wind'.

Certain abnormal pulse configurations occur under seasonal conditions. Generally speaking, the pulse may be wiry during spring, overflowing and strong during summer, superficially located during autumn, and deeply located during winter. When these abnormal pulses occur during these seasons, they should be considered as normal configurations.

Abnormal Pulse Configurations

Generally speaking, abnormal pulses are reflected in the pulse rate and location, as well as in the pulse configuration. There are, all in all, 27 different types of abnormal pulses. The appearance of these pulses can help diagnose a patient's overall clinical pattern of diseases.

Here are eight of the most distinct pulse configurations.

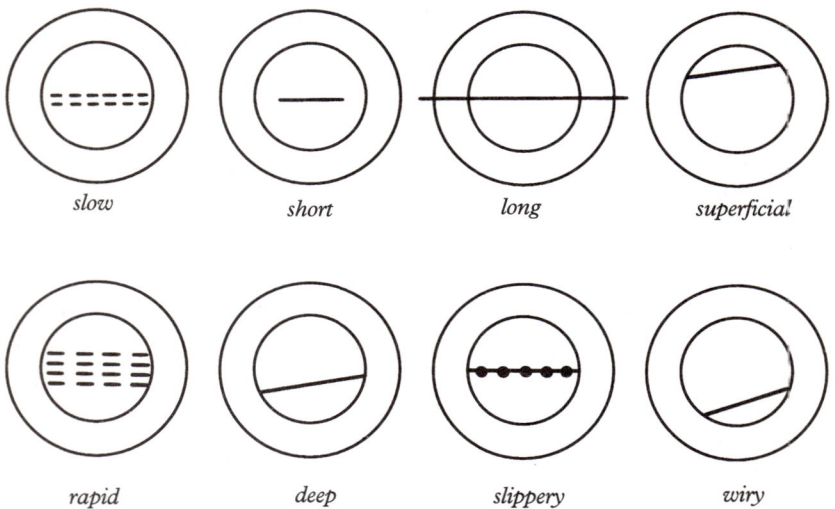

slow   short   long   superficial

rapid   deep   slippery   wiry

Diagrams of Various Pulse Patterns

Slow pulse — This is less that four beats per breath. This type of pulse may be felt among patients who have a cold clinical pattern where there is a deficiency of yang Qi. This pulse can also point to the accumulation of phlegm and blood stasis, when there is a slowing down of Qi and of the blood circulation.

Rapid pulse — This is more than six beats per breath. This pulse may be felt in hot clinical patterns when symptoms of fever or feverish sensations are felt.

Superficial pulse — This type of pulse may be felt just as the fingers are placed over the pulse. It is strong and clear when pressed lightly and becomes weak when pressed strongly. This pulse indicates an invasion by external pathogenic factors like wind heat or cold on the surface of the body.

Deep pulse — This may be felt only after applying heavy pressure upon the pulse. Ancient medical scholars often described this pulse as similar to a 'boulder or stone sinking towards the bottom of the water'. This type of pulse occurs in interior clinical patterns, whereby disease-causing factors have succeeded in weakening the body's anti-pathogenic Qi.

If the 'inch' segment pulses in both arms are deep, this indicates phlegm or mucus accumulation in the organ systems of the upper body, like the lungs and heart systems.

Long pulse — With this type of pulse, the whole breadth of the pulse seems to extend beyond the confines of the pulse's three regions. This may be due to a difference in height or build of the practitioner and patient or it can indicate an abundance of internal heat. If this pulse has a clearly defined configuration and is smooth in texture, and if the person has no abnormal signs and symptoms, it is a sign of good health and longevity.

Short pulse — With this type of pulse, the bar segment seems to rise while the two ends seem to descend, which gives the impression that the pulse is unable to 'fill in its place' among the three regions of the pulse. The movement of the pulse is uneven and short in duration with irregular missed beats. This pulse indicates a declining original Qi (see Glossary).

Wiry pulse — This is also referred to as a 'bow string pulse'. The pulse feels taut and forceful similar to the over-stretched strings of a drawn bow. It feels fixed in its location and quite smooth. This type of pulse indicates hyperactivity of liver yang.

Rolling or slippery pulse — This pulse flows smoothly and forcefully. The configuration is described as 'beads of pearl rolling in a porcelain basin' or a 'drop of water rolling on the blade of a lotus leaf'. This pulse indicates phlegm and mucus retention, as well as a sign of food retention (similar to symptoms of indigestion).

If this type of pulse is felt on the 'foot' region of the radial pulse and there are no other clinical signs and symptoms, then it is considered a normal configuration. When it is felt on the foot region of a woman's pulse and appears quite different from the configuration of the inch region then it is an indication of possible pregnancy.

STAGE TWO: ESTABLISHING CLINICAL PATTERNS

On the basis of data collected from the Four Examination Techniques, the TCM practitioner ascertains the specific clinical pattern of a patient. Because of the time factor, not all of the methods of examination described are used, but a thorough investigation of the patient's condition must nevertheless be conducted.

Usually, the main focus of examination is to establish the clinical pattern of the patient's chief complaint. This might be a cough, diarrhoea, insomnia, pain, headaches, wheezing, irregularities in normal cycles (e.g. menstrual irregularities, constipation), fatigue or sense organ dysfunction (e.g. loss of appetite, hearing deterioration, skin disorders).

A practitioner may detect, from information collected by the Four Examination Techniques, a clinical pattern that points to a pathological mechanism defined within the parameters of TCM but not obvious to the patient.

Verification of data is vital in establishing a clinical pattern. This is especially true in examining the tongue and the pulse. For example, some patients have the habit of brushing off their tongue coat every morning when they brush their teeth. If this is not established through inquiry, then a false impression of the tongue coat may be gained and an error in diagnosis can occur.

TCM Conceptual Templates

After analysis and verification of data have been made, TCM conceptual templates are used to structure the patient's signs and symptoms.

In the several millenia of TCM development, numerous conceptual templates have been developed and used to construct clinical patterns. Most of these conceptual tools have been developed by integrating ancient philosophical thought with the practice of TCM. Some of these philosophical thoughts originated from several ancient Chinese philosophical schools, such as the Yin and Yang, Taoist, Confucian, Five Elements philosophy, Chan and Mohist schools.

A template originally was a pattern outlined on a thin piece of wood used by a stone mason to cut a stone to a designed shape. I have taken the idea of templates from David Turnbull (1993) who advanced the notion of templates as models or patterns used to shape stones which were assembled to construct the Gothic cathedrals during medieval times in Europe. Through the medium of templates it was possible to organise large numbers of men to build these cathedrals. Also, through these templates, knowledge and skill about the building of Gothic cathedrals were passed on to the succeeding generation of builders. From this context I have extended David Turnbull's definition of templates to that of 'conceptual templates' which are also exemplars, used in TCM to assemble complicated signs and symptoms of diseases into clinical patterns.

The most common conceptual templates used in TCM diagnosis are: The Eight Principal Patterns (Ba Gang Bian Zheng); The Patterns of Pernicious Influences (Liu Yin Bian Zheng); The Patterns of the Six Divisions (Liu Jing Bian Zheng); The Patterns of Internal Organ Disharmonies (Zang Fu Bian Zheng); The Patterns of Four Stages (Wei Qi Ying Xue Bian Zheng); The Patterns of Acupuncture Channels (Jing Luo Bian Zheng).

The Eight Principal Patterns and the Patterns of the Six Divisions were developed by Zhang Zhong Jing, the father of TCM, during the Han Dynasty (206 BC–AD 220). The Eight Principal Patterns orders signs and symptoms into four contradictory phenomena of yin and yang; hot and cold; deficient and excess, and external and internal patterns.

The Patterns of Four Stages was developed by proponents of the Warm Febrile Diseases School during the Ming Dynasty (1368–1644). They re-ordered the signs and symptoms of fever-related diseases into four stages. It is a further development of the Pattern of Six Divisions pioneered by Zhang Zhong Jing.

The Patterns of Pernicious Influences orders the signs and symptoms of diseases into six categories according to the excesses of external climatic changes: wind, cold, summer heat, fire, damp and dryness.

The Patterns of Acupuncture Channels and the Patterns of Internal Organ System Disharmonies structure the signs and symptoms of various diseases according to disharmonies in the normal functioning of the acupuncture channels and the internal organ systems with which they are associated.

The use of one or a combination of these TCM conceptual templates in ordering and structuring the data gathered from the Four Examinations Techniques will establish the site of the disease (bing wei); its stage of development (bing shi); its cause (bing yin); and its mechanism (bing ji). Using the various criteria set by these TCM conceptual templates, multitudes of clinical signs and symptoms can be ordered and structured into almost 2000 clinical patterns. Below, clinical signs and symptoms are structured using the criteria set by the TCM conceptual templates of the Eight Principal Patterns.

The Eight Principal Patterns BA GANG BIAN ZHENG 八钢辨证

With the conceptual template of the Eight Principal Patterns, clinical signs and symptoms assembled through the Four Examination Techniques may be classified into the eight dual, contradictory patterns of internal or external, hot or cold, excess or deficient and yin or yang.

Internal or external patterns indicate the general site of the illness as well as the progression of the illness. Hot or cold patterns indicate the nature of the illness which may also determine which type of TCM discipline is best to employ, e.g. herbal, acupuncture or massage. Deficient and excess patterns indicate the balance of power between pathogenic Qi (disease-causing factors) and the anti-pathogenic Qi (body's capacity to resist them). The yin and yang patterns classify signs and symptoms into a broad context. Generally speaking, external, excess and hot patterns are yang patterns while internal, deficient and cold patterns are yin patterns.

External Patterns *Biao Zheng* 表证

External patterns are signs and symptoms which point to a disease or illness which is on the exterior of the body. The development of an illness displaying external patterns is still slight and superficial. Its assembled signs and symptoms are the following: an aversion to cold with fever, headaches and pain in other parts of the body, blocked nostrils and/or running nose, a thin white coating on the tongue and a superficial pulse.

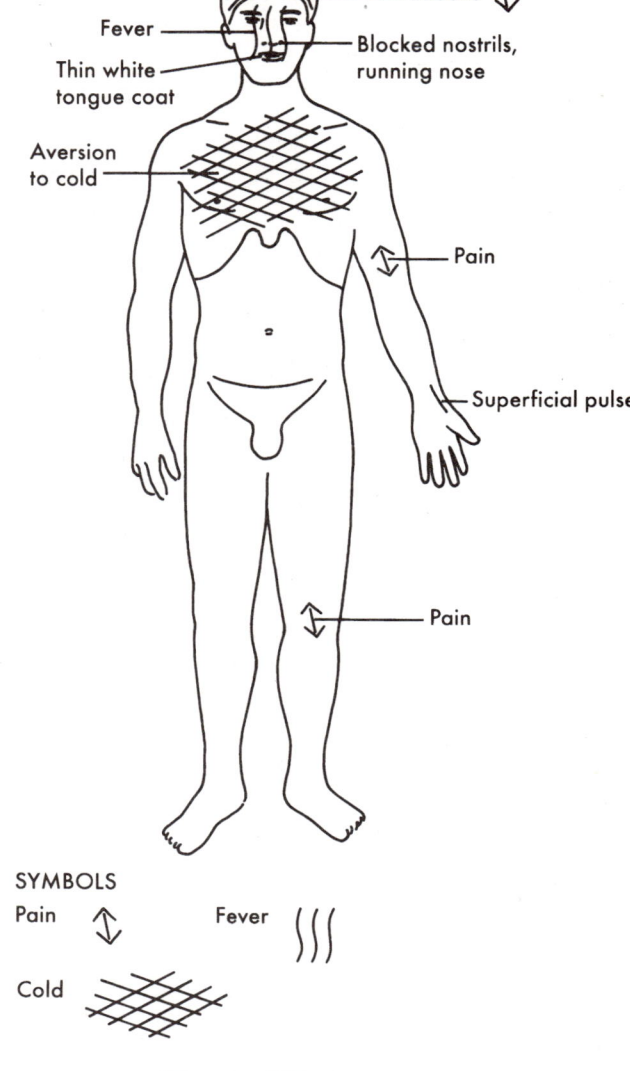

Headache

Fever

Blocked nostrils, running nose

Thin white tongue coat

Aversion to cold

Pain

Superficial pulse

Pain

SYMBOLS

Pain

Fever

Cold

External Pattern

Internal Patterns *Li Zheng* 里证

Internal patterns are signs and symptoms which appear when external patterns have not been dealt with properly and the illness has progressed from the exterior of the body to the internal (organ systems), hence the name. The signs and symptoms of this clinical pattern varies depending upon which internal organ system is affected.

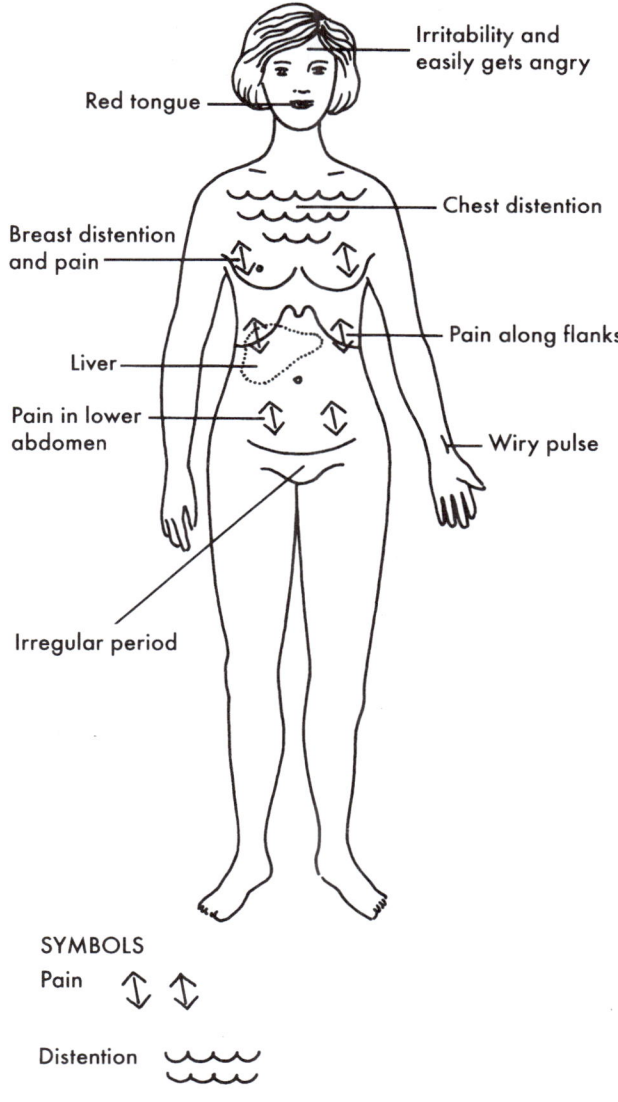

Internal Pattern

Cold Pattern *Han Zheng* 寒证

This clinical pattern may be the result of a pathogenic cold-factor invasion or the attenuation or weakening of bodily functions. The signs and symptoms are: pale facial colour, an aversion to cold alleviated by warmth or heat, a desire to lie in bed and not move around, cold extremities, an absence of taste in the mouth and no thirst, loose bowel motions, a tongue with a white moist coat, a deep and slow pulse.

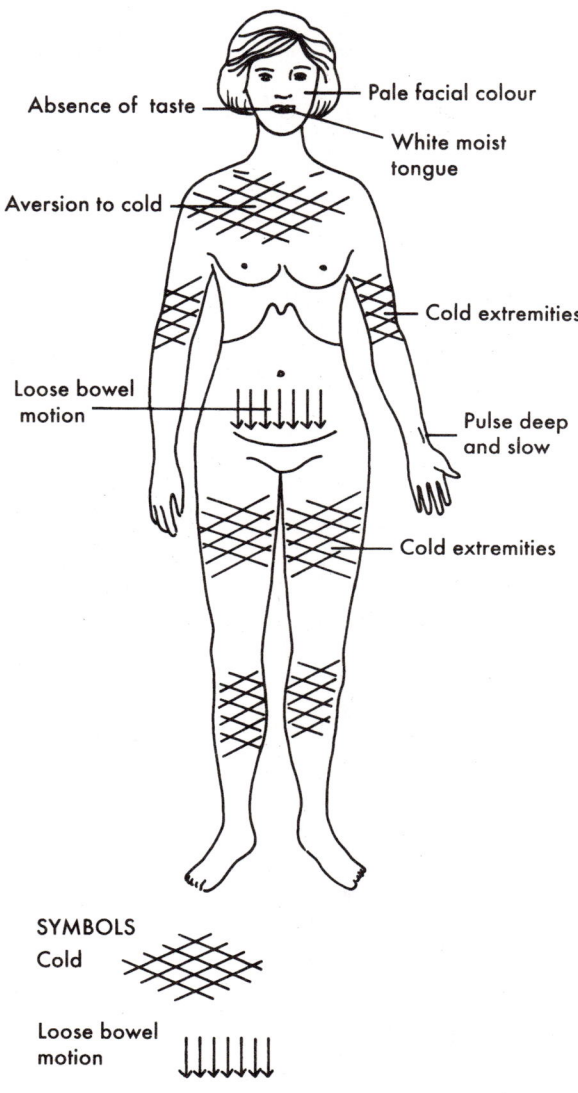

Cold Pattern

Hot Pattern *Re Zheng* 热证

This clinical pattern arises from either a pathogenic heat-factor invasion or from hyperactivity of body functions. The signs and symptoms are the following: flushed face and redness of the eyes, fever or feeling of heat alleviated by cold drinks or exposure to cold temperature, a sensation of heat in the body's extremities, thirst alleviated by a cold drink of water or juice, dark yellow urine released in short spurts, a red tongue with yellow coat and dry, a strong, rapid and wide pulse.

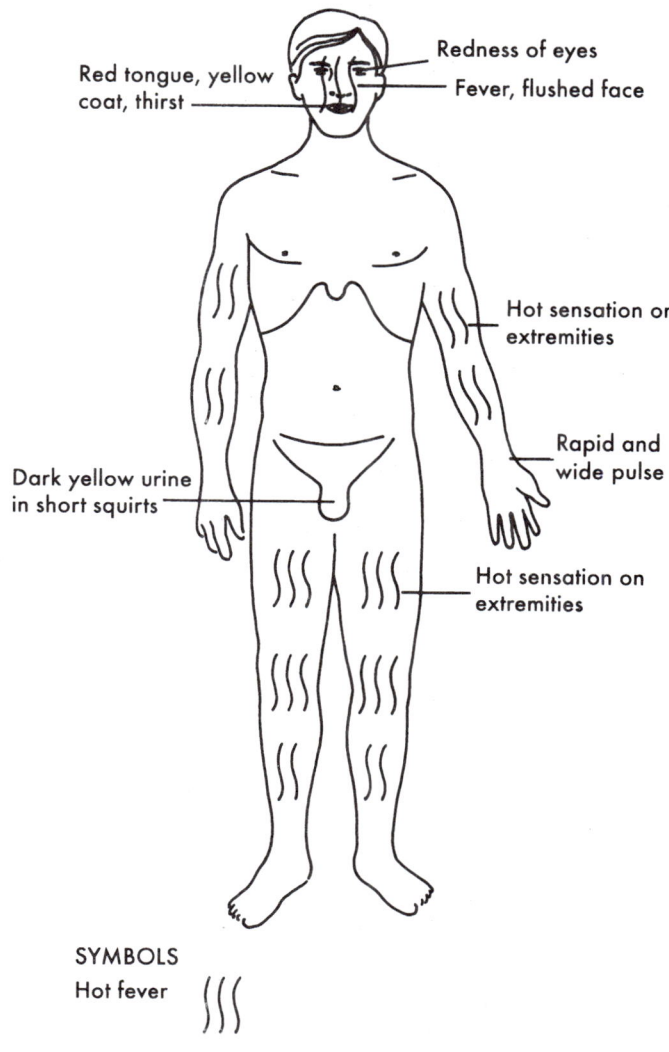

Red tongue, yellow coat, thirst

Redness of eyes

Fever, flushed face

Hot sensation on extremities

Rapid and wide pulse

Dark yellow urine in short squirts

Hot sensation on extremities

SYMBOLS
Hot fever

Hot Pattern

Deficient Pattern *Xu Zheng* 虚证

Deficient patterns arise from a weakening of the body's overall resistance to disease-causing factors (pathogenic Qi). The signs and symptoms are: shortness of breath, lack of spirit and vigour, physical debility, spontaneous sweating or night sweats, uncontrollable urination, loose bowel motions, a pale tongue, a weak and thin pulse.

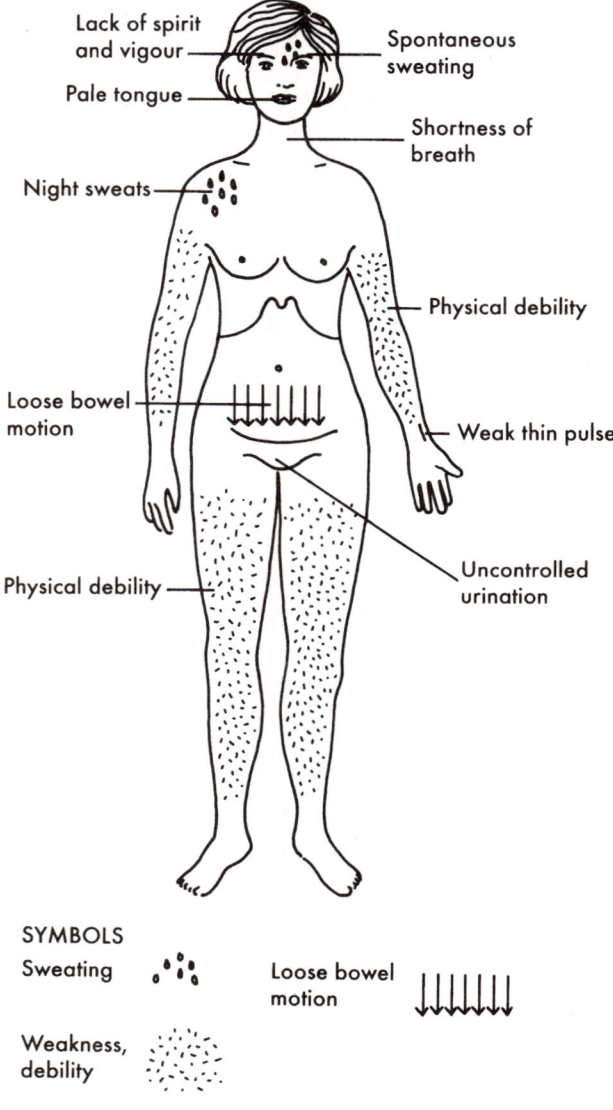

Lack of spirit and vigour

Spontaneous sweating

Pale tongue

Shortness of breath

Night sweats

Physical debility

Loose bowel motion

Weak thin pulse

Physical debility

Uncontrolled urination

SYMBOLS

Sweating

Loose bowel motion

Weakness, debility

Deficient Pattern

Excess Pattern *Shi Zheng* 实证

This clinical pattern arises due to the dominance of the pathogenic Qi (disease-causing factors) over the anti-pathogenic Qi (overall body resistance). The signs and symptoms are: rough breathing, irritability, distention of the chest and abdomen, pain with aversion to palpation or touch, a feeling of blocked urination, dry stool or constipation, red tongue with thick dirty coat and a strong pulse.

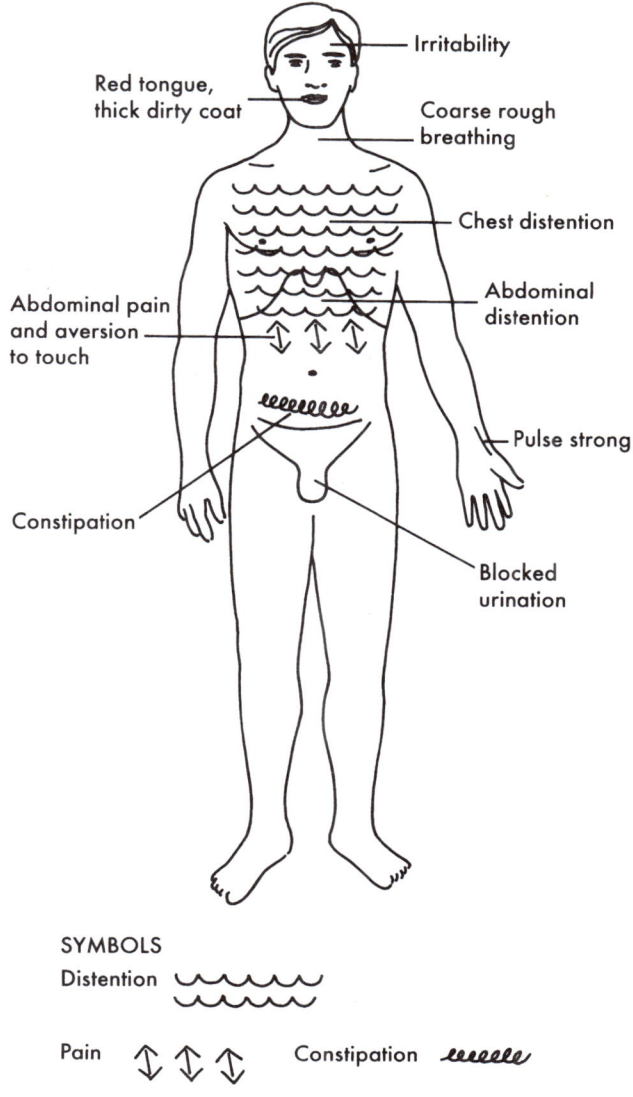

Excess Pattern

Yang Pattern *Yang Zheng* 阳证

A yang pattern is a broad category which may encompass external, hot and excess patterns. The signs and symptoms are hyperactivity of body functions, a strong body resistance to pathogenic Qi on the exterior of the body. Disease manifestations are of the hot type characterised by an active and sensitive bodily response.

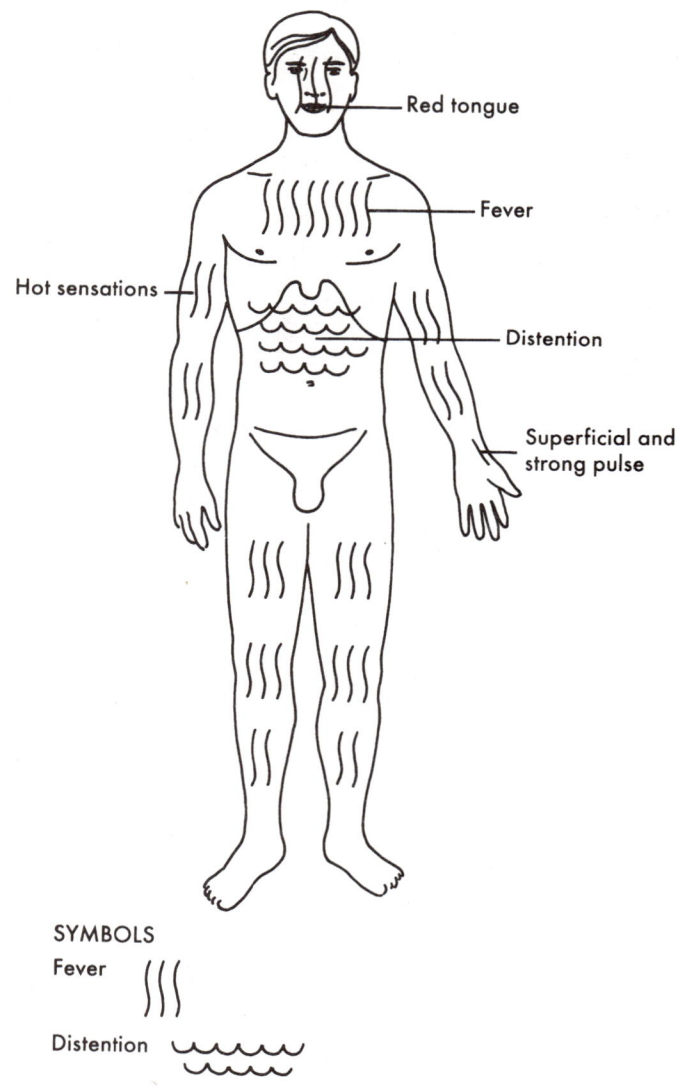

Red tongue

Fever

Hot sensations

Distention

Superficial and strong pulse

SYMBOLS

Fever

Distention

Yang Pattern

Yin Pattern *Yin Zheng* 阴证

Yin pattern is the opposite of yang pattern. Signs and symptoms are a weakening of bodily functions, a deficient resistance to pathogenic Qi (i.e. manifestations of cold, inhibited, descending and weakened body response), and an internal disease-causing factor.

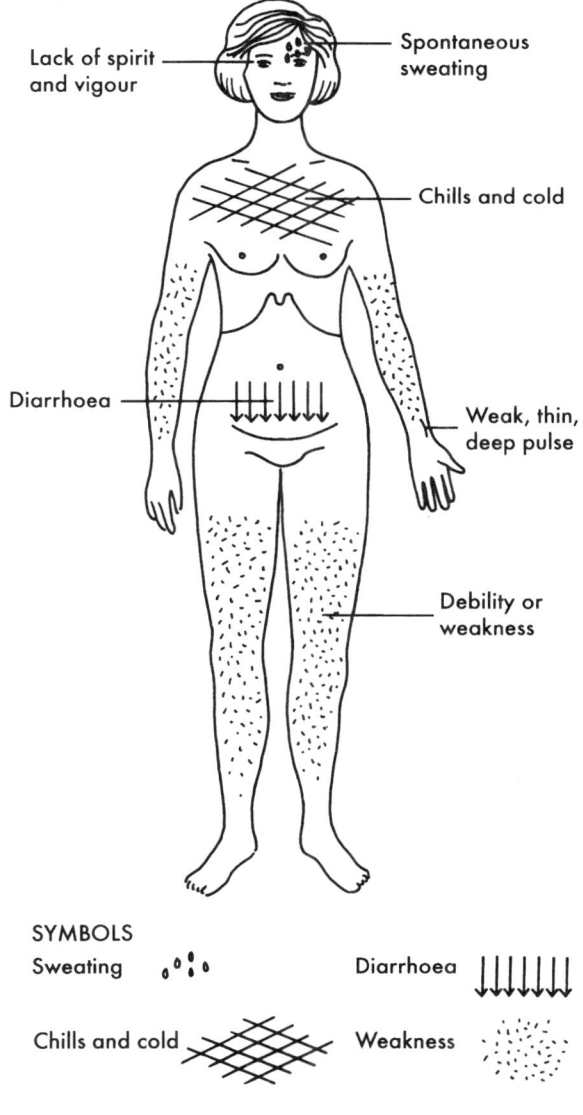

Yin Pattern

Establishing the Therapeutic Principle, Method and Formula

The clinical pattern of a patient reflects both the signs and symptoms of and the cause of illness or the 'li' 理 pattern. 'Li' is the principle which explains why and how these clinical patterns come about. 'Li' is a Chinese philosophical concept which has a variety of meanings in different contexts. In this context, it means — as defined by Han Fei Zi, a Han-dynasty legalist philosopher — the 'culture which explains how things come about'.

Once the 'li' of a particular clinical pattern has been established, the stage is set for deciding on a particular therapeutic method or 'fa' 法 for dealing with this clinical pattern.

Based upon a specific clinical pattern, the practitioner will decide whether to deal with the root or underlying cause of the illness or to deal with the more acute or pressing conditions.

There is a choice of eight therapeutic methods: diaphoretic (han fa); emetic (tu fa); downward (xia fa); dispersing (xiao fa); mediating (he fa); warming (wen fa); clearing (qing fa); and tonifying (bu fa). Generally the diaphoretic method is used to deal with an exterior clinical pattern; the dispersing method is used for getting rid of accumulated mass or tissue brought about by the stagnation of blood or Qi; the mediating method for a clinical pattern in which the disease-causing factor is halfway between the exterior and interior regions of the body; the emetic and downward methods for excessive and internal clinical patterns; the clearing method for hot clinical patterns; the warming method for cold clinical patterns; and the tonifying method for deficient clinical patterns.

The diaphoretic, dispersing, emetic, downwards and clearing methods can be broadly categorised as sedating or reducing methods; while the warming methods are categorised as reinforcing or tonifying methods. The mediating method is neither sedating nor reinforcing.

Once the therapeutic method has been chosen, then a therapeutic strategy called a formula or 'fang' 方 is used to deal with a particular clinical pattern.

The formula may be a herbal decoction, a series of acupuncture points or a repertoire of massage techniques (tuina). It may also include specific advice to the patient. There are thousands of herb formulae and hundreds of acupuncture and massage formulae to choose from. The fang or formula may also be a combination of therapeutic disciplines, e.g. a mixture of acupuncture, herbs and tuina.

'Yao' 药 refers to individual harmonising remedies which together make up a formula. They may be herbs, acupuncture points, an individual massage technique or some individual advice.

The old Chinese script for 'yao' 药 is made up of symbols for bells and a drum set on a wooden platform with a Chinese radical script representing plants and herbs on top. So 'yao' in its ancient meaning refers to the 'orchestration of music' (Weiger, 1965) which can provide pleasure and joy just as properly used medicines restore health and pleasure in living.

In TCM practice, one can encounter specific clinical patterns for which no specific formula is set down. In this case, the practitioner concocts an individual formula which may include a wide range of herbs, food and medicinal substances, acupuncture points and massage techniques.

In conclusion, while the practice of TCM may be summed up by the four Chinese characters of 辨证论治 (bian zheng lun zhi), which means proposing treatment principles in accordance with the clinical pattern, it can also be generalised into the four Chinese characters of 理法方药 (li fa fang yao) which translates as 'choosing individual remedies for a formula on the basis of the established therapeutic method and principle'.

Case Study

The following is an account of a case of severe diarrhoea treated by the author in 1990 in Australia. This example demonstrates how the TCM practice of proposing treatment principles in accordance with clinical patterns can be used successfully.

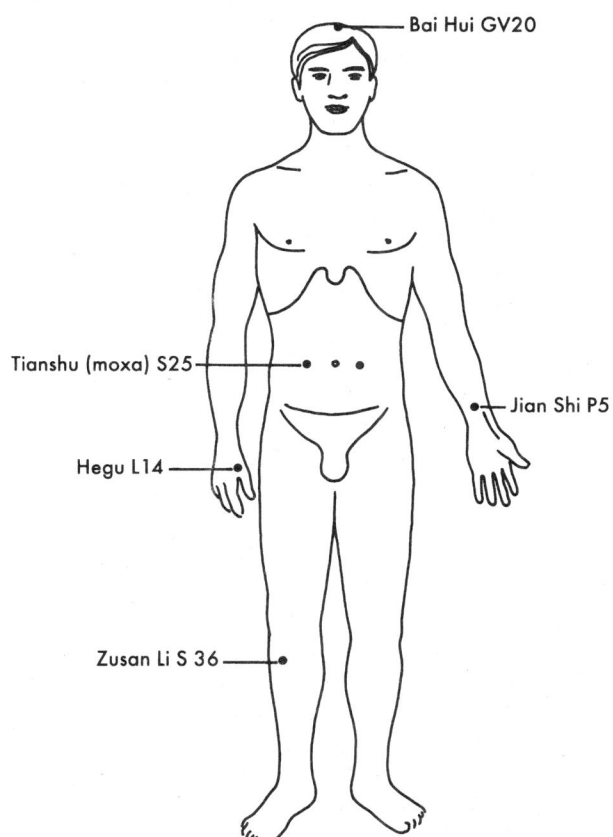

Case History: Acupuncture Points Used

Paul, male, 47 years old, computer programmer

Main complaint: Diarrhoea (12–30 times a day) for the past couple of weeks after eating some sausages bought from a butcher shop. Loose watery bowel motion. Patient has lost 8 kg as a result. No history of severe diarrhoea. Patient taking Lomotil tablets and antibiotics. Patient also complains of coldness on the back.

Examination: 16/2/90. Pulse: deep and taut. Tongue: red and moist. Patient looked very tired and had low-pitched voice. Facial complexion is pale; with enhanced blackness around the eyes. Sleep is not good due to anxiety and frequent visits to the toilet. Inquiry also revealed that patient had acupuncture from another practitioner a couple of years ago to quit smoking.

Treatments: 16/2/90 Acupuncture was administered to the patient using the following acupuncture points:

1. Bai hui GV 20 (top of the head).
2. Tian shu S 25 (both sides of the navel). Burn a piece of moxa stick on handle of the needle.
3. Jian shi P 5 (just above the wrist crease on the inner side of both forearms).
4. He gu LI 4 (at junction of thumb and index finger of both hands).
5. Zusanli S 36 (just below both knees). Burn moxa stick on handle of the needle.

19/2/90 Patient came for next consultation and therapy. Upon inquiry, the patient said that he had felt very good right after the first treatment and the diarrhoea had stopped on same day. He reported that he slept the whole afternoon on the day of the acupuncture treatment up to the early afternoon of the following day. He is now having only two bowel motions each day and it is not loose. Similar acupuncture treatment was administered to the patient.

Subsequently, the patient had three more acupuncture treatments (administered once every second day), using the same acupuncture points and technique. By the time of the last consultation and therapy, the patient was back to a healthy state.

Discussion: The choice of acupuncture points, as well as the technique of moxibustion, was made on the basis of the presenting clinical pattern of the patient when he came on the first day of treatment.

The above data were gathered on the basis of observing, listening, inquiring and taking the patient's pulse. Then the conceptual template of the Eight Principal Patterns was used in structuring the presenting signs and symptoms of the patient. It was deduced that it was a predominantly yin clinical pattern. This is evidenced by symptoms and signs of watery diarrhoea (a downward yin symptom), loss of weight, low-pitched voice, pale facial complexion with enhanced blackness around the eyes, deep pulse and a moist tongue. Diarrhoea also points to a disharmony within the internal organ systems of the spleen and large intestines. It is therefore not an external pattern. The deep pulse also indicates an internal pattern. Loose bowel motions, a low-pitched voice, loss of weight and a pale facial complexion also point to a weakened anti-pathogenic Qi which reflects a deficient pattern.

The patient's main complaint was diarrhoea and this was brought on by eating the sausage bought from the local butcher shop. The sausage was probably not properly cooked or had gone off. Food goes off easily during summer. This information about the food came after inquiring about the history of the main complaint and how it came about.

The sausage affected the transporting function of the intestinal system, which resulted in a build-up of pathogenic dampness followed by loose bowel motions. The loss of body fluid and inability of the transporting systems to absorb food and water brought about the dramatic loss of weight, the pale facial complexion and enhanced blackness around the eyes. This in turn led to a deficiency of Qi which accounts for the deep pulse, tiredness and low-pitched voice.

This clinical pattern pointed to a deficiency of the yang Qi and a build-up of dampness in the body. This is the li of the clinical pattern. The therapeutic method or fa used to deal with this clinical pattern is to tonify the yang Qi while dispelling the dampness to eliminate diarrhoea.

In the acupuncture point formula chosen, bai hui GV 20, jian shi P5 and he gu LI 4 were used to dispel dampness. The burning of moxa on zusanli S 36 helped to boost the Qi while burning the moxa on tian shu S 35 helped to dispel dampness.

The rapid favourable response of the patient after the first treatment shows that the treatment principle (lun zhi) used corresponded to the clinical pattern (zheng hou).

Therapeutic Action GONG XIAO 功效

Every clinical pattern requires a particular therapeutic approach. A cold clinical pattern requires a hot therapeutic approach; a hot pattern requires a cold therapeutic approach; a deficient pattern requires a tonifying approach; an excess pattern requires a sedating approach and a yang pattern requires a yin approach.

In the course of the long evolution of TCM's therapeutic disciplines, practitioners have effectively employed thousands of combinations of foods, acupuncture points and massage techniques in dealing with a multitude of clinical patterns. Eventually, these 'recipes' were recorded, classified and categorised into what is referred to as their 'gong xiao' or therapeutic action.

'Gong' 功 means an achievement, result, skill or work. This is a Chinese character which combines the script for 'work' 工, with the script for 'strength' 力. 'Xiao' 效 means to imitate or to follow the example of, so 'gong xiao' means a result which has to be imitated or a result which is reproducible.

Every herb or herb formula, acupuncture point or acupuncture points formula, every individual or combined massage technique formula, each food or combination of foods has a therapeutic action which addresses a particular clinical pattern. For example, one of Ginseng's therapeutic actions is to tonify a deficient Qi in a deficient clinical pattern. A reinforcing needling manipulation or a kneading massage of the accupuncture point 'Three Leg Regulator' S 36 has a tonifying Qi therapeutic action. Eating an apple has a similar therapeutic action.

The therapeutic action of these individual remedies has been determined and confirmed by prolonged use. It is thus the work of the TCM practitioner to 'imitate' or 'reproduce' these 'effects' by adopting the appropriate remedy with the appropriate therapeutic action for a specific clinical pattern. If the clinical pattern is redressed and the illness is cured, then the treatment principle is proven to be correct. However, if the clinical pattern does not respond to the therapy, then the practitioner has to reassess the case to determine the correct diagnosis and remedy.

In recent times, clinical researchers in China have been re-ordering or translating signs and symptoms of various clinical patterns into a biomedical pathological system of diagnosis, i.e. a modern medical system of diagnosis. Diseases are first diagnosed in accordance with their biomedical parameters, i.e. blood, urine, blood pressure, neurological tests etc. Following this, their clinical pattern is defined in accordance with the classification of signs and symptoms according to TCM diagnosis. Based upon this combined diagnostic method, acupuncture, herb, food and massage are used to deal with a clinical pattern. Subsequently, pathological testing is employed to objectively measure the efficacy of the treatment.

For this reason, a significant amount of TCM literature now includes biomedical parameters, such as 'lowering blood pressure' or 'deactivating viral or bacterial micro-organisms' in defining the therapeutic efficacy of certain herbs or acupuncture points.

TCM DISCIPLINES

I have presented in this book the main disciplines of herbal medicine, food therapy, acupuncture, tuina (therapeutic massage), and nurturing life, and TCM's system of diagnosis which are the disciplines best known and widely practised in the West.

In China, TCM disciplines are far more differentiated and specialised. In general, TCM disciplines may be broken down according to the following categories: clinical practice, research and education.

Within the clinical practice category, TCM disciplines may be divided into two major areas: internal medicine (nei ke 内科), and external medicine (wai ke 外科). Internal medicine may be compared to the area of general Western medicine, but in TCM 'internal' also has the added meaning of treating diseases which affect the internal organ systems. It also is used in the sense of boiled decoctions being administered 'internally'.

'External medicine' or 'wai ke' is sometimes loosely and inappropriately translated into the English term 'surgery'. While historical accounts of surgical operations are documented in Chinese medical history, this type of medical practice did not evolve. Instead of the scalpel, the Chinese evolved the ancient external technological device of the acupuncture needle.

External medicine or 'wai ke' therefore refers to those therapies applied to the exterior of the body, such as acupuncture, tuina, cupping etc., as well as therapeutic herbal ointments, oils or essences applied to acupuncture points or channels on the surface of the body.

In addition, external medicine covers those diseases which manifest themselves on the body's exterior such as skin disorders, malignant and benign tumours, sprains, fractures and dislocations.

TCM disciplines may also be differentiated according to illness and patient types. Under this system of categorisation TCM disciplines may be differentiated into external, internal, gynaecological or female diseases (fu ke), men's illnesses (nanke, which deals with male sexual dysfunctions like impotency), paediatrics (er ke), eye diseases (yan ke) and ear, nose, throat (er bi hou ke) disciplines.

TCM disciplines may also be classified according to therapy types, i.e. acupuncture, herbal medicine, food therapy, nurturing life, tuina, Qi Gong, traumatology (shang ke) and integrated TCM-Western medicine.

Traumatology is a TCM discipline which evolved out of warfare and martial arts in China, and includes tuina massage techniques and manipulation techniques to treat sprains, fractures and dislocations. Spinal manipulation techniques akin to those of osteopathy and chiropractic are also included in the discipline.

Integrated TCM -Western medicine (zhong xi yi jie he) is a discipline which evolved from combining TCM and Western medical practice.

Research work encompasses all the above mentioned clinical disciplines. In addition, there is the discipline of ancient textural research which looks into the thousands of ancient medical texts and TCM basic theory research which looks into the historical, etymological and philosophical aspects of TCM theory.

TCM education puts a premium upon clinical training. Hence, the above clinical disciplines are all included in TCM university curricula. Aspects of Western medical disciplines, such as anatomy, physiology, histology and biochemistry which blend with the TCM body of knowledge, are also included in the curriculum.

• C H A P T E R   I I •

A BRIEF HISTORY OF TCM
中医简史

THERE ARE THREE CRITICAL FACTORS WHICH CONTRIBUTED TO THE HISTORICAL construction and development of the TCM body of medical knowledge. These were: the continuous and uninterrupted evolution of practice and experience in recognising and treating diseases for more than four thousand years; the use of philosophical concepts to order and organise the construction of this practice into a flexible, systematic and coherent body of knowledge; and the use of a unique pictographic language to accurately encapsulate and record TCM's evolutionary development.

The following presentation of the history of TCM concentrates on the main strands of the philosophical weaving of its practice from antiquity to the present.

With regard to the linguistic factor, certain relevant points need to be established. Among the many ideographic languages in the world, Chinese to date is one of very few which has remained ideographic or pictographic and resisted any move towards conversion to an alphabet or romanisation. This is a phenomenon which has baffled many scholars and linguists.

Chinese linguists have explained the resilience of the Chinese ideogram in terms of its great capacity for plasticity, or ke suo xing, and its possession of 'virtual life', or xu huo xing, to represent itself directly. Accordingly, while retaining its original meaning, the Chinese character can adapt and change its meaning to the requirements of a new era, continually absorbing new culture, thinking and consciousness.

An example is the evolution of the character for 'king' or wang 王. Currently, this script is written with three horizontal lines with one vertical line connecting the three. During the time of the Shang Dynasty (1660–1100 BC), the character for king was inscribed on the oracle bones as 𠆢, which represents the image of a man standing on the ground, overweening, arrogant and considering himself unexcelled in the world. However, during the time of the Song Dynasty (AD 960–1279), the philosopher Wang An Shi in developing his philosophy of 'oneness between heaven and man' (tian ren he yi) re-defined and re-wrote the meaning of 王. The three horizontal lines represent heaven, man and earth, while the vertical line which connects the three is the king.

EARLY PREHISTORIC ORIGINS OF TCM

As a body of practical medical knowledge, TCM originates from the birth of Chinese civilisation, dating back to the primitive Stone Age. As society moved forward materially, socially and economically, so did the practice of medicine.

During the primitive period of food gathering and the subsequent periods of hunting, domestication of animals, agriculture, mining and iron smelting, the medicinal values of herbs, animal by-products and minerals were discovered. These activities constituted the embryonic stage in the development of the Chinese materia medica or ben cao 本草.

In the course of innumerable repetitions of gathering, hunting, tasting, using and eating food, plants and minerals, the early Chinese worked out which substances were edible, poisonous or therapeutic. The edible substances alleviated hunger and provided nutrition, the poisonous induced dizziness, vomiting, increased urination, diarrhoea or sweating; while the therapeutic were found to alleviate some ailments. These reactions led to a primitive cognition of certain 'inclinations' or attributes of substances.

Initially, individual herbs were used indiscriminately and randomly to deal with certain ailments. Later, when combinations of herbs were used to deal with more complicated conditions, this process became more systematised. Eventually, this evolved to become the use of a group of herbs in a formula to deal with clinical patterns.

With an increased availability of herbs, food and animals, the use of fire, the development of pottery, the fermentation of wine and improved culinary skills, the technique of herb decoction evolved. During the Stone Age period, stone needles known as 'bian' 砭 stones emerged. These were used for tapping body surfaces, incising or pricking boils and abcesses. The bian stone eventually evolved into animal bone, pottery shard, bamboo and finally into the modern-day metallic disposable stainless steel acupuncture needle.

With the discovery of fire, it was accidentally discovered that applying heat to the abdominal region relieved abdominal pain and other conditions. This led to the development of the primitive technique of 'hot pressing' or yun 熨, the precursor of moxibustion. Accidental rubbing, pinching and kneading of certain parts of the body was found to relieve certain ailments or pain. Hence with repeated experience, the art of massage or tuina evolved. Communal and tribal dancing gave rise to the later development of the various traditional physical exercises of Qi Gong and Tai Chi.

SHAMANISM Wu Yi 巫医

During antiquity, especially during the latter part of the Shang Dynasty (1600–1100 BC), the shaman or 'wu yi' emerged as a powerful authority, who by prayers, incantations, sacrificial offerings to the Gods and spirits, ridded people of their illnesses.

During this period, the Chinese character for medicine or Yi was written differently, as 醫 The upper part of the character represents a hand which is grasping arrows to drive away the evil spirit, while the lower portion is the character 'wu' 巫, which represents two shamans or 'priest-doctors' at work.

One of the methods used to relate to the Gods and spirits was divination or 'zhan pu' 占卜. This entailed burning tortoise shells or the scapula bone of a large mammal (later known as oracle bones). The fortune of a person was foretold according to the shape of the cracks on these materials after burning.

During this time, illness was thought to be an independent phenomenon caused by the power of an evil spirit or ancestor. If the shaman determined that this was the case, he offered prayers and devised techniques to have the evil spirit or ancestor leave. The patient and the family members also made sacrifices to the Gods, amends for past mistakes, appeased the ancestors and made a vow to satisfy and get rid of the evil spirits. If the illness became serious and developed into near death, this was taken as a sign that the Gods did not forgive the patient.

Oracle Bones

From the archaeological remains of the Yin Dynasty ruins, approximately 160,000 oracle bones used by shamans were left for posterity, with 323 pieces containing the inscriptions of more than 20 illnesses.

During ancient times, illness or disease was referred to as 'ji' 疾. The inner portion of this character 矢 is an arrowhead, while the outer portion 疒 is a radical indicating diseases. The word 'ji' in Chinese means suddenly falling ill as if being struck by an arrowhead. It can also mean lying in bed with beads of sweat emerging from the body or leaning in discomfort against a chair.

Some of the illnesses written in the oracle bone style of writing — the earliest type of character writing in China — were classified in accordance with their site, i.e. head, ear, eye, abdomen, tooth, foot etc. Some inscriptions appear to describe symptoms like tinnitus, diarrhoea or insomnia. Hence, the earliest records of the concepts of illnesses in China were encoded in these oracle bone inscriptions.

THE PHILOSOPHICAL ROOTS OF TCM

Over twenty-one hundred years, from antiquity (2105 BC) up to the Warring States period (475–221 BC), medical knowledge accumulated incrementally. This was followed by half a millennium (475 BC–AD 24) of summing up and construction in accordance with the philosophical framework of that time.

The Warring States period is known as the period in which ancient philosophers and a 'hundred schools of thought contended'. It was during this time that various philosophical schools like Confucianism, Taoism, Mohism, the Legalists, and Logicians flourished and influenced almost all spheres of life, including culture, art, politics, medicine and astronomy. The three philosophical concepts which significantly contributed to the construction of the TCM knowledge system during this time were those of yin and yang, the Five Elements or wu xing 五行 and the Qi.

Although the concept of yin and yang and the Five Elements originated during the earlier time of the Western Zhou Dynasty (1100–771 BC), it was during the Warring States period that it merged into one conceptual framework.

These two concepts provided a broad structure for making sense of the natural world without resorting to shamanism and divination.

The earliest meaning of yin and yang was in reference to the sun. That side facing the sun is yang, while that aspect against the sun is yin. Subsequently, these meanings were extended so that all things were classified into having a yin or yang natural attribute or tendency, e.g. sun (yang), moon (yin), heaven (yang), earth (yin), day (yang), night (yin), fire (yang), water (yin), hot (yang), cold (yin), etc.

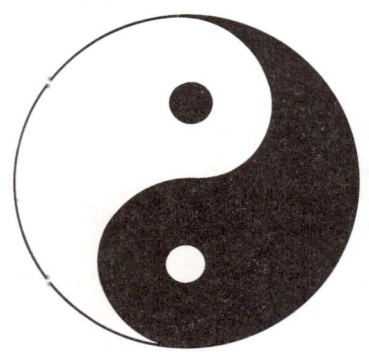

Yin and Yang Symbol

According to the concept of yin and yang, the phenomenon of change in nature is a product of the mutual interaction, opposition and transformation between the dual yin and yang aspects of things. The ebbing of yin leads to a flow in yang, and the peak of yin leads to transformation into its opposite yang, e.g. peak of night (yin) leads to day (yang) and vice-versa.

The concept of the Five Elements refers to wood, fire, earth, metal and water. Originally, these were no more than the basic materials upon which nature is constituted. However, on the basis of the attributes or natural tendencies of each of these elements, i.e. the moistening qualities of water; the smouldering qualities of fire; the bending and extending qualities of wood; the sound-producing qualities of metal and the capacity of the earth to grow plants and other living things, complicated inter-relationships were formed among them. There is a mutual generating relationship between the five elements, i.e. water generates wood; wood generates fire; fire generates earth; earth generates metal and metal generates water. There is also a mutual

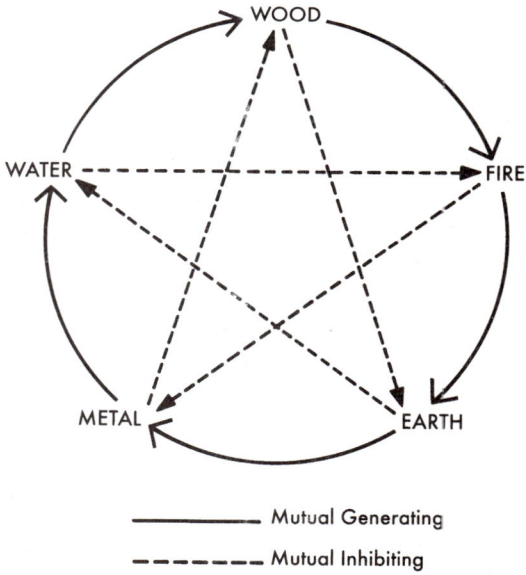

Five Elements - Wu Xing

inhibiting relationship between the five, i.e. water inhibits fire; fire inhibits metal; metal inhibits wood; wood inhibits earth and earth inhibits water.

Yin and Yang and the Five Elements Categorised According to their Associations

		YANG		YIN	
Element	*Wood*	*Fire*	*Earth*	*Metal*	*Water*
season	spring	summer	long summer	autumn	winter
weather	windy	hot	damp	dry	cold
colour	green	red	yellow	white	black
flavour	sour	bitter	sweet	pungent	salty
visceral organ system	liver	heart	spleen	lungs	kidneys
emotion	anger	happiness	pensive	worry	fear
hollow organ system	gall bladder	small intestines	stomach	lower intestines	urinary bladder
body form	tendon	blood vessel	muscles	skin	bones
sense organ	eyes	tongue	mouth	nose	ears
massage technique	pluck	push	grasp	knead	press

These interactions were further extended to explain complicated natural, life, medical, disease, therapeutic, and even social phenomena.

Another major philosophical concept was the concept of the Qi (pronounced 'chee'). Qi originally referred to 'floating clouds', the 'breath and the atmosphere between heaven and earth'. Mythology has it that the universe emerged from a 'cloud of mist' amidst a great cosmological confusion. The light and pure yang Qi ascended to become heaven while the heavy course thick yin Qi descended to become earth.

During the Warring States period, philosophers considered that all visible things in the universe originated from an invisible Qi, which itself was a product of a mixture of faint objects that cannot be identified or touched. It was not until the period of the Eastern Han Dynasty (AD 25–220) that Qi was identified by Taoist philosophers as the primary origin of the universe as well as all the myriad of things in it. They contended that it was the most basic substance from which the cosmos was made up and that all visible things originated from Qi and were the product of its multitude of transformations. According to the Taoists, Qi is the 'very minute particles in continuous motion, the deep spring and the motive force in the transformation of things'.

The philosophy of yin and yang, the Five Elements and Qi, as well as other Taoist philosophical concepts of the time, provided the conceptual tools with which medical scholars were able to erect and order the construction of the TCM body of knowledge.

FORMATIVE YEARS OF THE TCM BODY OF KNOWLEDGE (475 BC–AD220)

The TCM body of knowledge as we now know it took form from the Warring States period (475–221 BC) through the Qin Dynasty (221–207 BC) and on into the Han Dynasty (206 BC–AD 220). These 700 odd years coincided with the beginning of 2500 years of feudalism.

It was during this period that the four great classics in TCM were written. These were the two volumes of the *Yellow Emperor's Canons on Medicine* (黄帝内经) (the first volume is *Questions and Answers* and the second volume, *Canon on Acupuncture*), *Shen Nong's Materia Medica* (神农本草经) and the *Treatise on Febrile and Other Diseases* (伤寒杂病论).

Canons on Medicine HUANG DI NEI JING 黄帝内经

The *Yellow Emperor's Canons on Medicine* laid the foundations of TCM. Of unknown authorship and reputed to have been written over several generations, the two volumes comprise over 140,000 classical Chinese characters, 36 sections and 162 chapters. Subsequently annotated by hundreds of medical scholars, it is a comprehensive medical classic which is still seriously studied by current TCM students and practitioners.

On the basis of repeated medical practice and observation, the *Yellow Emperor's Canons on Medicine* made use of the concepts of yin and yang, the Five Elements and the Qi to explain the normal structure and functioning of the human body. This resulted in the development of the concepts of the Visceral and Hollow Organ Systems and the Acupuncture Channel System (zang fu jing luo xue shuo 脏腑经络学说).

The visceral organ systems are those of the heart, liver, spleen, lungs and kidneys, while the hollow organ systems are those of the gall bladder, stomach, large intestine, small intestine, urinary bladder and triple energiser (see glossary).

The visceral organ systems include the anatomical physical organs and their functional manifestations, which are systematised according to ancient philosophical principles, including yin and yang and the Five Elements.

As an example, the heart system or 'xin' 心, which is the most important visceral organ system, is compared to a monarch. Apart from controlling blood flow, it houses the spirit or shen 神 and is considered the main organ system governing mental activities, including memory, thought, sleep, consciousness and emotions. Most of the present-day known functional manifestations of the central nervous system are attributed to the heart system. The heart corresponds to the element of fire, the emotion of happiness and is connected by the heart acupuncture channel network, to the tongue and face (the barometers of the heart condition) and the small intestine system.

The interactions between these organ systems are also set by the system of the Five Elements, as is shown by the process of transformation of fluid substances when taken orally. Quoting from the classic, 'Fluid substances that are taken orally are digested in the stomach organ system. The constitutional essence derived from the fluid is spread to the spleen organ system which in turn sends it to the lungs'. (The spleen, which corresponds to the element of earth generates or promotes the lungs which correspond to the element of metal.) 'Through the dispersing and descending function of the lung organ system, the water passageway is cleared, which paves the way for the waste water to be sent to the urinary bladder'. (Lungs, which correspond to the element of metal, generate the urinary bladder, which corresponds to the element of water.). 'This process of spreading the fluid then allows the constitutional essence of the water to be distributed throughout the body and flow to the five organ systems.' Note how the elements and organ systems in the Five Elements Table on page 35 are arranged according to their mutual generating inter-relationships, i.e. wood generates fire, which generates earth, which generates metal, which generates water; similarly a pathway is defined from the liver to the heart to the spleen to the lungs to the kidneys and from the gall bladder to the small intestine to the stomach to the large intestine to the urinary bladder.

In addition to the elucidation of the body's physiology with the aid of philosophical tools, the classic also named 311 diseases under 44 categories which included conditions we would presently associate with fevers, parasitic diseases, diabetes, nephritis, hepatitis, diarrhoea, haemorrhage etc. At this stage, however, systematic disease diagnosis in accordance with the clinical pattern of signs and symptoms had not yet been adopted. The canon basically employed the four techniques of examination: observing, listening and smelling, inquiring and palpation. Pulse diagnosis was made by pulse taking of the wrist, head, neck, legs and feet.

The second volume of the canon comprehensively dealt with acupuncture, including the channels, points and needling techniques. Certain herbs and herb formulae were mentioned, although not systematically.

Clinical Patterns — a System of Diagnosis

The *Treatise on Febrile and Other Diseases*, written by the father of TCM, Zhang Zhong Jing (circa AD 150–219) established the clinical method of 'proposing treatment principles in accordance with the clinical pattern' or bian zhen lun zhi 辨证论治. This laid the foundation of TCM clinical principles and methodology.

Zhang Zhong Jing, on the basis of the *Yellow Emperor's Canon on Medicine*'s concept of visceral and hollow organ systems and acupuncture channels, developed a method of categorising the complicated signs and symptoms of fever-related diseases and other illnesses into clinical patterns or zheng hou 证候.

According to Zhang, each clinical pattern represents a stage in the progressive development of the disease. These typical clinical patterns were ordered into what is referred to as the stages and sub-stages of the Six Divisions: three yang (greater, brighter and lesser) and three yin (greater, lesser and terminal).

For each clinical pattern, proven effective herbal formulae or other remedies were tailored and prescribed. About 113 herbal formulae were tailored for each clinical pattern. A system for tailoring a therapeutic principle, a therapeutic method, a herbal formula or an individual remedy for a particular clinical pattern was developed.

The Earliest Pharmacopoeia

Shen Nong's Materia Medica, the earliest pharmacopoeia in China, pioneered the classification of herbs in accordance with their four Qi attributes (hot, warm, cool, cold), five flavours (pungent, sweet, sour, bitter, salty) and their therapeutic actions. It laid the theoretical foundations for the use of herbal medicine. Three hundred and sixty-three herbs and other medicinal substances (252 herbs, 67 animal by-products and 46 mineral substances) were classified into three levels of categorisation with their therapeutic actions directed at more than 170 types of illnesses and clinical patterns.

PERIOD OF RAPID GROWTH OF THE TCM BODY OF KNOWLEDGE (AD 265-960)

With the laying of its theoretical foundations, TCM practice entered a period of rapid growth and development. This 700-year period is characterised by the further development of radial pulse-taking, diagnosis by clinical patterns, improved techniques in herbal processing and the setting up of a comprehensive Imperial Academy of TCM. Contacts with other systems of medical knowledge also started during this period.

Wang Shu He (AD 201–280) was the first medical scholar in China to systematise the use of radial pulse-taking in diagnosing a clinical pattern. In his *Classic on the Pulse* he described in detail 24 different pulse patterns using the depth, length, feel and rate of the various segments of the radial pulse. At the same time, he closely linked the pulse with the clinical pattern and the therapy required.

In the year AD 610, the first specialised book to systematise diseases and clinical patterns was written by another medical scholar, Chao Yuan Fang, who was an Imperial physician. The work was organised by the Imperial Medical College under the sponsorship of the Imperial government.

His *General Treatise on the Origins of Diseases and Clinical Patterns* 诸病源候总论 recorded 1720 clinical patterns of diseases covering internal, external, gynaecological, paediatric etc.

In AD 657, the Imperial government commissioned the compilation of the first official pharmacopoeia in China, the *Revised Materia Medica* 新修本草. This pharmacopoeia included illustrations and descriptions, and the therapeutic actions of 844 medicinal substances. Alchemy, which became the vogue in China during this time, gave impetus to the development of various methods of processing herbs and other medicinal substances.

During the Tang Dynasty (AD 618–907), specialisation in TCM was reflected in the writing of books in such specialised fields as acupuncture, paediatrics, massage, food therapy, traumatology, obstetrics and medicinal substance processing.

The rapid growth and development of the TCM body of knowledge led to the setting up of the Highest Imperial Medical Office or Tai Yi Shu in AD 624.

This official body, which was the highest medical body in the country, was also a TCM training college for practitioners destined for the Imperial Court. At its peak, the office employed 340 personnel. After studying the *Yellow Emperor's Canon on Medicine, Classic on the Pulse* and *Shen Nong's Materia Medica*, the students underwent apprenticeship or internship for several years in the various departments of internal medicine, acupuncture, materia medica and massage.

During this period, Buddhism reached China and so began the co-existence of Buddhism, Taoism and Confucianism. Buddhism had a significant influence in the development of TCM.

Through the written medical classics, TCM began to reach countries surrounding China such as Japan, Korea and Vietnam, and it spread as far as the Middle East via the Silk Road trade route.

PERIOD OF TCM ACADEMIC FERMENT AND BIRTH OF VARIOUS SCHOOLS (AD 960-1368)

This period covers four centuries, from the Song Dynasty (960–1279) to the time when China was ruled by the Mongol Yuan Dynasty founded by Kublai Khan (1271–1368).

It was during the Song Dynasty that movable type printing was invented which effectively hastened the dissemination of TCM knowledge in the country and increased academic ferment. The first bronze acupuncture model was designed and used in the Imperial Medical College. The *Revised Materia Medica* was reprinted with revisions and additions of more medicinal substances.

Important books on herb formulae were published during this time. The *Taiping Sacred and Benevolent Formulae* 太平圣惠方 compiled and presented 16,834 various herbal formulae, together with the clinical patterns and diseases that could be treated in accordance with the principle developed in the *General Treatise on the Origin of Diseases and Clinical Patterns*.

In the area of clinical-pattern diagnosis, the causes of diseases were classified into three major divisions: internal causes (excessive emotions of fear, sadness, happiness etc), external causes (triggered by excesses of seasonal and weather changes, e.g. wind, cold, heat, dryness, dampness), and other causes (diet, injury from animal and insect bites, physical injuries etc).

In clinical medicine further specialisation also evolved. From the Jin Dynasty (1115–1234) to the time of Kublai Khan's rule during the Yuan Dynasty, academic ferment set into TCM circles. Medical scholars started to question the wisdom of only relying upon the classics to solve present day-illnesses. They pointed out that 'the old medical classics cannot cure all of today's illnesses'. This unleashed a debate among medical scholars which resulted in the birth of several schools of thought in TCM.

Four main academic schools emerged with their respective advocates and representative classical works. These were: the Cold and Cooling School; the

Expelling and Purgation School; the Tonifying The Earth (Spleen Organ System) School and the Nourishing the Yin School.

The Cold and Cooling School mainly came from North China where the weather is very cold and where fever-related illnesses were rampant. They advocated the use of herbs with cold and cooling attributes to deal with these fever conditions and they stressed the importance of acknowledging a patient's constitution in diagnosing clinical patterns.

The Tonifying The Earth School advocated that the spleen system be of predominant concern when dealing with every condition. They contended that 'hundreds of illnesses come from internal afflictions of the spleen organ system'.

The Expelling and Purgation School opposed the predisposition to always tonify the patient. Instead, they advocated the use of diaphoretic (sweating), clearing (as in clearing pathogenic heat) and emetic (vomiting) therapies.

Finally, Nourishing the Yin School saw the tonification of the Yin constitutional essence as necessary due to the fact there is 'always excess yang and deficient yin'.

THE BIRTH OF A NEW SCHOOL IN DIFFERENTIATING CLINICAL PATTERNS (1368–1911)

The Ming (1368–1644) and Qing Dynasties (1644–1911) were the last of the feudal dynasties in China. During this period, before the founding of the first republic in China by Dr Sun Yat Sen in 1911, there were three outstanding developments in the field of TCM. These were the birth of a new method of diagnosing clinical patterns, the publication of the first major work on materia medica and the arrival of Western medicine.

During the sixteenth century, major epidemics, which were then referred to as 'wen yi' 温疫, broke out in many parts of China. During the 500 odd years of Ming and Qing Dynasties, 138 epidemics, which killed thousands of people, were recorded.

The old 'Six Divisions' method of diagnosing and treating fever-related clinical patterns, which had been developed during the Han Dynasty, now proved inadequate. Medical scholars realised an incongruity when they increasingly observed that epidemics were occurring seasonally and that the clinical manifestations were different to those expounded in the 'Six Divisions'. As a result, a new school, the Warm Febrile Diseases School 温病派 emerged with Wu You Xing as its main proponent.

This school recognised that fever-related illnesses were not only caused by seasonal factors or excesses of wind, cold, damp or heat etc. They re-ordered the symptoms and signs of fever-related illnesses into the Pattern of Four Stages, defined as the outer (wei), next (qi), inner (ying) and blood (xue) phases of invasion. The illnesses were believed to be a type of Qi which entered the body through the nose and mouth. New herbal formulae and therapeutic approaches were adopted to accommodate this fresh approach.

It was also during this period that human variolation 'dou zhen' 痘疹 was developed as a method of immunisation against infectious diseases. One method involved the practice of healthy people inhaling the infected scab fragments of smallpox rashes as a means of disease prevention. Historians have recognised this practice as being the forerunner to the smallpox vaccination developed by Jenner in 1796.

Herbal Pharmacopoeia by Li Shi Zhen

In 1578 the most comprehensive pharmacopoeia, the *Compedium on Materia Medica* 本草钢目 was published by an Imperial Medical College medical scholar, Li Shi Zhen (1518–1593). Written over a period of 30 years and comprising more than 1,500,000 characters and over 800 Chinese reference materials, it described 1892 herbs and 11,000 herbal formulae.

During this time, the Imperial Medical College was subdivided into 13 specialities, including gynaecology, oral diseases, traumatology, febrile diseases, acupuncture and massage. In 1822, however, acupuncture received a setback when the Manchu (non-Han Chinese) Court banned its use, for it was deemed to be unsuitable for the Manchu nobility.

Early contacts between TCM and Western Medicine

The sixteenth century marked the coming of European Christian missionaries, who influenced the development of TCM by introducing the Chinese to some Western medical knowledge of the time. Foremost among these missionaries was Father Matteo Ricci, who brought with him books on anatomy and physiology. During this time, TCM books on pulse reading, acupuncture and materia medica were translated into English, French and other European languages.

A BIG TESTING TIME FOR THE TCM BODY OF KNOWLEDGE (1839–1949)

The period from the Opium War (1839–1842) until the establishment of the People's Republic (1949) was a difficult time for the development of TCM in China. In the past, TCM was able to co-exist with other foreign philosophical influences like Buddhism. However, the influx of a very different Western scientific medical system backed by a modern European political, military, economic and cultural power created a crisis for TCM.

Some medical scholars faced with a different knowledge system thought that going back to the TCM classics was the best option, while others, who had received their education in Western medicine and science from the missionaries, started to look down on their own indigenous medicine. Yet another group that had studied Western medicine and science on their own saw the strong and weak points of both systems of knowledge and advocated a combination of the two. These medical scholars were eventually named the TCM Western Medicine Combined School.

One of the most notable proponents of this school was Zhang Xi Chun, (1860–1933), author of *Records of TCM and Western Medicine in Combination*. In this book, pharmaceutical drugs, such as aspirin, natrium salicylicum, sololum, magnesium sulfurium and aether, were classified according to their Qi attributes and flavour, and used in accordance with varying clinical patterns used in the TCM system of diagnosis.

Despite the birth of this school, the crisis in TCM continued and culminated in the introduction of a resolution in 1929 in the Chinese Parliament to 'ban the old medicine in order to sweep away the obstacles to the development of medicine, health and pharmacology'. This resolution included the banning of TCM educational schools, TCM registration and the practice and promotion of TCM. Although the resolution was successfully opposed by TCM practitioners and their supporters so that it did not become law, it nevertheless marked a decline in the practice of TCM at the time.

TCM UNDER THE PEOPLE'S REPUBLIC (1949 – PRESENT)

When the People's Republic was established in China in 1949, one of the earliest policies it enunciated was the integration of TCM with Western medicine. This entailed the setting up of TCM research and educational institutions. It also necessitated the standardisation of academic and clinical training in both TCM and Western medicine, with a TCM component included in Western medical training and a Western medicine component in TCM courses. Old TCM practitioners were to be trained in Western medicine, and practitioners of Western medicine in TCM. Today, practitioners of both TCM and Western medicine are registered as medical practitioners in China.

In terms of academic development, the present government in China advocates co-existence between the TCM school, the Western medicine school and a new school of integrated TCM and Western medicine. The latter uses the 'modern, western, scientific perspective and methodologies' to research TCM's traditional practice and concepts. One fruit of this integration was the 1970s breakthrough in the use of acupuncture anaesthesia for surgical operations.

TCM ETHICS Yi De 医德

During its long history, TCM evolved a system of ethical principles covering the cultivation of inner character, attitude to medical skills and the relationship with colleagues, and with the sick and the dying.

Central to these ethical values is the cultivation of the inner character, or 'ren' 仁: human-heartedness, benevolence or kind-heartedness. It is one of the five Confucian norms which include righteousness or yi 义, propriety or li 理, wisdom or zhi 志 and faith or xin 信. 'Ren' or human-heartedness, which is the 'virtue that unites men to men' (Weiger, 1965), is cultivated from within and is manifested through one's actions.

A TCM practitioner must empathise with the pain which the patient experiences and share his anxieties, without thought of his or her own selfish desires. One ancient Chinese medical scholar stated that a TCM practitioner 'who is not kind-hearted should not be trusted'. Another scholar stated 'It is all right for one to study medicine to save the dying. However, it is not acceptable to study medicine just for one's selfish gains'.

A Ming-dynasty (1368–1644) medical scholar, Gong Ting Xian, compiled the 'Ten Important Points That a TCM Doctor Must Observe' which sets out the responsibilities of a practitioner to her- or himself and to the patient. He also drew up the 'Ten Important Points That a Patient Must Observe' which outlined the responsibilities of a patient to her- or himself and to the practitioner. Although these points are very prescriptive, they set out in clear terms some ethical rules which guided the symbiotic relationship between the practitioner and patient during those times. Some of these points still serve as a reference for proper conduct in the current practice of TCM in China.

'Ten important points that a TCM doctor must observe'

1. Keep one's inner human-heartedness. Be good at giving people advice. Be charitable to the public, which will bring profound gratitude.

2. Be good at observing the Confucian ethics. Such a doctor will be a treasure to succeeding generations, will refer to the classics and will be clear in her or his principles.

3. Be good at taking the pulse to differentiate exterior and interior clinical patterns. When the fingers are 'clear', severe illness can be dealt with appropriately.

4. Clarify the origin of the illness so one can dare judge the outcome in terms of life or death. If practitioners reach this level of skill, then they are considered a specialist in the field.

5. Be knowledgeable of the seasonal movement of the Qi, which will make clear the sequence of the year. In this way, tonifying or sedating or using warm or cold remedies can be done in accordance with the right timing.

6. Be clear about the acupuncture channel systems. Avoid mistakes in diagnosing illnesses. One must understand the visceral and hollow organ systems before one can be considered a Bian Que (famous ancient Chinese doctor).

7. Know the Qi attributes and flavours of herbs to establish the right formula for an illness. If one is not clear about the warm and the cold Qi attributes, then one can harm and endanger life.

8. Have the ability to prepare and process herbs, and be meticulous in the use of heat in processing them. Heat should be neither too strong nor weak.

9. Do not be too envious and jealous and do not treat people differently on account of kinship. Heavenly principles will then make themselves clear.

10. Do not make huge profits from people. Make sure you maintain 'human-heartedness'. While there are differences between the rich and the poor, do not practise double standards in prescribing remedies to them.

'Ten important points that a patient must observe'

1. Choose a brilliant doctor. One cannot afford not to be careful in this regard, for life or death depends on it.

2. Be willing to take medicinal remedies which will rid illnesses. The foolish person who always procrastinates, only delays treatment.

3. The earlier the treatment the better. Early treatment is easier to deal with. The metaphor, 'if one steps upon the frost, then one knows that winter is coming' is a way of saying that if one is aware of having symptoms of an illness and is not treated as early as possible, then more severe health consequences will follow.

4. Stop all chamber (sexual) activities when one is sick. If one goes against this, then even a skilled doctor will have no way to deal with it.

5. Guard against extreme anger. Anger brings about fire from which one may be difficult to save.

6. Stop all wishful thinking. Nurture the tranquillity of the spirit. Once anxieties have passed, the spirit turns pleasant.

7. Regulate eating and drinking. There should be rhythm and regularity. Over-eating can lead to indigestion.

8. Be prudent about daily routine. Socialising must be lessened. A little bit of manual work will heal the body's deficiency.

9. Do not believe in the shaman, as this can lead to serious consequences. Heresy and lies only confuse people.

10. Do not put too much value on cost. Why put too much value on it? 'May I ask the gentleman, is there anything more precious than the treasure of life?' from Gong Ting Xian (circa 1600) (Ming Dynasty, 1368–1644) *Bringing Back Spring from Ten Thousand Illnesses* 万病回春 in *Famous TCM Doctors During Past Dynasties: Discussions on Ethics* (1983). 历代明医医德, Hunan Science & Technological Publishing House, Hunan, China pp. 209–211.

• C H A P T E R   I I I •

TCM OUTSIDE CHINA
中医在国外

IN AUSTRALIA TRADITIONAL CHINESE MEDICINE HAS A HISTORY OF ALMOST ONE and a half centuries. The initial transfer of this medical knowledge system (mainly herbal medicine) from China transpired through the medium of the Chinese migrants who arrived during the middle of the nineteenth century in search of gold.

As Chinese settlement grew in areas such as Bendigo, Ballarat and Melbourne, the practice of TCM also developed. By 1867, there were 50 Chinese herbal medicine practitioners on the Victorian goldfields of Ballarat, Bendigo and other places. This compares well with 25 registered practitioners of Western medicine in 1866 (Loh, 1985). By 1911 herbal remedies were being sold to non-Chinese in Victoria. Herb bottles were labelled in English with clear directions for administration. By 1925, practitioners of Chinese herbal medicine in Victoria organised and collected petitions to oppose the introduction of a bill in parliament which limited the dispensing of medicinal herbs to pharmaceutical chemists. A section of the petition reads: 'We record our belief that orthodox medical practitioners do not possess a monopoly of the only proper method of curing disease' (Loh,1985) and went on to point out that TCM has been practised for thousands of years. Over 6000 people signed the petition (a substantial number at that time) and this led to the withdrawal of the bill in the Victorian parliament.

The practice of traditional Chinese herbalism has ebbed and flowed in Australia. Events such as the world wars and domestic events in both Australia and China have affected the supply of herbs and the flow of migration. The starkly perceived differences between TCM and Western medicine, as well as the dominance of the European colonial-scientific medical system of knowledge have also affected and still affect the ebb and flow of TCM practice in Australia.

During the 1970s, acupuncture provided the impetus for another 'flow' of TCM practice in Australia The breakthrough in acupuncture anaesthesia in China, as shown to the world by satellite television during the Nixon visit, generated interest about this ancient TCM discipline. In the 1970s government-sponsored health insurance provided full acupuncture cover for patients, paradoxically, of registered Western medical practitioners.

During the 1980s a great shift in attitude occurred towards medicine. There was a move away from a paternalistic monolithic orthodox medical system towards consumer-oriented medical pluralism, with the flourishing of a vast range of alternative medicines, including naturopathy, homeopathy, traditional

Chinese medicine (particularly acupuncture), chiropractic and osteopathy. Private alternative medical colleges, as well as professional acupuncture organisations, were set up in various cities. Standards of acupuncture ethics and practice were introduced and developed.

In the early 1990s government-accredited university degrees in traditional Chinese medicine and acupuncture were first offered. Currently, three universities in Australia offer these courses. Private colleges also run courses in acupuncture, tuina and herbal medicine.

It is noteworthy to point out that TCM practitioners come not only from the ethnic Chinese community but also from the Anglo-Celtic, Italian, Greek, Vietnamese, Filipino and other communities, reflecting the wide interest in TCM among different ethnic groups.

The decade of the 1990s ushered in another 'high' in the practice of TCM. In 1992, practitioners and representatives of 16 TCM, acupuncture and herbalist organisations all over Australia met in Melbourne to form a unified association, the National Traditional Chinese Medicine Liaison Committee (NTCMLC). They developed *Guidelines For A National TCM Curriculum At Tertiary Level (Australia)* which established and laid down the basic tertiary educational standards for institutions teaching TCM in the country.

Subsequently, TCM practitioners lobbied the federal government for a registration of qualified practitioners. During the 1993 Australian federal elections, the then federal Health and Community Services Minister, the Honourable Brian Howe, expressed his support for the registration of TCM practitioners in Australia in a letter to the Victorian Committee Chair of the National TCM Liaison Committee. He said 'I am happy to assure you of my support for Chinese medicine and acupuncture and for the registration of practitioners in these areas on public health and safety grounds.'

In response to this commitment from the Australian Federal Health and Community Services Minister, the National TCM Liaison Committee, which represents 16 associations throughout Australia, put a submission before the Health Minister's office calling for the introduction of federal legislation to register TCM practitioners. It proposed a self-funded registration board to be recognised by each State, which would consist of ten TCM practitioners, a Western doctor, a lawyer, a consumer representative and a federal health department representative. There still remains much lobbying to be done by practitioners and consumers before TCM practitioner registration eventually becomes a reality.

A DIALOGUE BETWEEN TCM AND WESTERN MEDICINE

To have meaningful dialogue between the two medical systems, an understanding of the history and practice of both is essential. Here follows a basic introduction to Western medicine.

The practice of Western science-based medicine has been through more than two thousand years of development, dating back from the time of Hippocrates (460–379 BC). Its systematisation as a knowledge system shifted from the vast expanse of several areas in the present Middle East and Western Europe and hence was nurtured by the linguistic and cultural backgrounds of these areas. During its development, it went through the four stages of 'library medicine', 'bedside medicine', 'hospital medicine' and finally the present 'laboratory medicine' (Ackerknecht, 1982).

Hippocratic medicine ushered in what is referred to as 'bedside medicine', which gives priority to the examination of presenting clinical symptoms. 'Library medicine', during its domination by the monks and Arab scholars of the Middle Ages, leaned heavily on the classical Greek texts. 'Hospital medicine', with the emphasis on correlation between lesions and symptoms, emerged during the eighteenth century. 'Laboratory medicine', which emphasised the integration of laboratory findings with clinical observations, began in the second half of the nineteenth century.

In the long history of Western medical practice, technoscience provides the important ingredient for the structuring of its medical knowledge system. (Current science philosophers view science as a knowledge system closely linked to society and vice versa and see no dichotomy between science and technology. They see both as an extension and embodiment of the other. Hence the use of the term 'technoscience'.) The experimental method, localisation of diseases (from organ, tissue, cell, genes etc), physics, chemistry, the microscope, the stethoscope, the laboratory and the micro-worlds all contributed to the unique science-based system of Western medical knowledge as we know it today.

TCM and Western science based medicine began its process of dialogue at the time of Matteo Ricci's sojourn to China in the sixteenth century. This dialogue has, to date, resulted in a non-dominant, largely dualistic system of medicine in China and the dissemination of TCM knowledge internationally. However in countries outside of China, science-based medicine is the dominant system of medicine, a situation which has led to the marginalisation of other systems of medicine which are not based upon that culture and tradition of science, for example indigenous systems, Chinese medicine, homeopathy, naturopathy, chiropractic etc.

With an increased awareness of other medical systems and a growing realisation of the diagnostic and therapeutic limitations and escalating costs of science-based medicine, consumers are increasingly raising questions about freedom of choice with regards to their health needs. Consequently there is an increasing demand for alternative or complementary systems of medicine including traditional Chinese medicine.

Set in this context, there is a need to internationally reinvigorate the dialogue between TCM and science-based Western medicine begun by Matteo Ricci over 500 years ago.

Some mistakenly argue that before it can be accepted as a system of medicine in the West, TCM must first prove itself to be 'scientific'. They contend that all the herbal formulae, acupuncture points, massage techniques etc. must first pass the systematic, foolproof and rigorous requirements of scientific validation, i.e. experimentation, double-blind trials, etc.

In China some TCM researchers are taking this route of subjecting aspects of TCM knowledge and practice to 'scientific' standards normally used to test Western science-based medical practice. In mid-1994, at an academic meeting of TCM practitioners in Melbourne, Australia, a TCM researcher from Sichuan province in the south-west of China spoke of the 'successes' they were reaping in their work of integrating TCM and Western medicine. He said, 'At present with the aim of making TCM scientific, the chemical composition of every single herb and formula is being isolated; all the TCM disciplines will be restructured into scientific disciplines, such as antomy, physiology, pharmacology, biochemistry etc. Because TCM will have a scientific language, you won't have to worry about it becoming accepted in the West.'

Unfortunately, if this brand of 'domination by scientism' (Farquhar, 1987) is achieved, the essentials of TCM will be lost for good. This will be a tremendous loss, not only to science, but to humanity itself.

TCM practice has a unique history, logic and method of knowledge generation. To use another knowledge system, like the Western science-based medicine, to judge its acceptability is inappropriate. It is akin to trying to make a round peg fit into a square hole. TCM, like all other systems of knowledge, can and should be allowed to stand on its own.

Hence there is an urgent need to find a better approach for conducting this dialogue between TCM and science-based medicine. We need an approach free from the dominating, narrow, dogmatic and decontextualising theories or 'isms'.

In Australia, the NTCMLC in 1992 used a unique exemplar in adopting Western medical disciplines in drafting a national TCM curriculum guideline for all universities and colleges wishing to offer TCM courses.

After looking at China's experience of integrating Western medicial disciplines into their own TCM curriculum, the committee selected aspects of Western medical disciplines which enhance the TCM core disciplines. For example, concepts of homeostasis in physiology, metabolism in biochemistry and the study of whole systems in anatomy, which complement TCM's perspective of balance, harmony and equilibrium, were integrated into the curriculum guideline.

The whole curriculum guideline was structured into five major divisions: General Subjects; Basic Medical Sciences; TCM Clinical Sciences; TCM Research and Methodology; and Supervised Practical Clinical Experience. About one-fifth of the entire curriculum guideline consists of Western medical sciences, which includes aspects of anatomy, physiology, pathology, histology and embryology, pharmacology, community medicine and Western medical diagnosis.

The drafting of this TCM curriculum guideline outside China marks a turning point in the continuing dialogue between TCM and Western medical science. First of all, it ensures the preservation of the essential ingredients of TCM practice. Furthermore, it demonstrates that the two systems of knowledge can work together for the common good.

TCM AND THE CONSUMER

Aware and proactive consumers of TCM

Being an aware TCM consumer means being a proactive, not a passive, patient. The success of a TCM therapy is not only contingent upon the diagnostic and therapeutic skill of the practitioner, it is also, to a very large extent, dependent upon the coordination and cooperation of an aware and knowledgeable patient.

When a patient is aware of the nature of TCM diagnosis, then he or she can coordinate with the practitioner to make sure that the relevant clinical data necessary for a diagnosis is made available. This may include data relating to menstruation, bowel motion, habits or lifestyle, some of which the patient may find embarrassing to divulge.

When all relevant data are provided to the practitioner, a clear clinical pattern is diagnosed and an appropriate therapeutic principle, method and formulae are determined. So a good patient-practitioner relationship is important.

Making the most of a TCM consultation

To make the most of a consultation with a TCM practitioner you should:

1. Try to see yourself as a whole person. Be aware of your body's rhythms, i.e. in sleeping, eating and defecating, and your lifestyle especially as it relates to the cycle of the seasons and weather changes. Try to see how your body's rhythms correlates with the onset and development of the signs and symptoms of your disease. This approach complements that of your TCM doctor who views illness as a product of disharmony among a body's organ systems as it interacts with the outside world.

2. As far as practicable, have a clear idea of your main complaint before seeing the practitioner. The main complaint is the sign or symptom which makes you suffer the most, i.e. headache, low back pain, dizziness, period pains, sleeplessness etc. It will help if you write this down before seeing your practitioner.

3. Describe your complaint in as much detail as possible. Clearly relate signs and symptoms which can be seen (colour, location on the body); heard (cough, wheezing, etc); touched (lumps) and smelt (body, urine or faeces

odour). This may include describing every sign and symptom, subjective feelings, onset and development of the condition, therapies undergone and responses to them. Show the practitioner any physical mainifestations of the disease such as skin rash, bruise, tender spot, swollen tissues etc.

4. Show your tongue in a relaxed and natural manner. Poke out and spread it as much as possible without overstraining the tongue muscles. Before the visit, avoid any food with food colouring, i.e. strawberry lollies, coloured chewing gum, cough lozenges or drinks, as these foods can affect the tongue's natural colour.

5. Avoid perfume, fragrant soaps, and body lotions as these may conceal significant body odours from the practitioner's investigation.

6. Avoid make-up, lipstick and other beauty aids as these may affect an accurate monitoring of facial colour or 'spirit'.

7. Avoid any strenuous physical activity immediately before a consultation as this may prevent an accurate pulse reading.

8. Bring along copies of any medical or diagnostic test reports and samples of any medication being used.

9. Avoid taking any alchohol or strong stimulants like coffee or tea two hours before a consultation.

Duration of TCM consultation and therapy

The nature of TCM consultation and therapy does not easily lend itself to what is referred to as 'assembly line' clinics. Since every case is treated individually, time is required to establish the clinical pattern and to tailor a specific individualised remedy.

It is of course possible to just have a consultation with a TCM practitioner without treatment but usually during the initial consultation the patient's history is taken, the clinical pattern established and the first treatment is given. This normally takes 30 to 45 minutes. Subsequent treatments take 20 to 30 minutes although acupuncture or tuina consultations tend to be longer, while herb consultations may be shorter.

Course of treatment

A TCM course of treatment varies according to the clinical pattern, the therapy used and the severity and chronicity of the condition. For example, therapy involving acupuncture, tuina or both for an acute lower back pain with no signs of bone fractures or dislocations may require a course of two to four treatments, structured either every day or every second day. However, a chronic lower back pain, with a specific clinical pattern would generally require a course of six to eight treatments, scheduled every second day.

Generally, with herbal therapy, once the herbs have been administered only one follow-up consultation is required. If the clinical pattern has not improved then the formula may be changed and checked at a subsequent consultation. However, if the patient is responding well, no follow-up is required for the course of herbs, which generally lasts for ten days.

Cost of consultation and health insurance

Some TCM and acupuncture professional organisations annually set the recommended consultation and therapeutic fee for their members. It is wise for the consumer to inquire about the professional fee before booking a consultation with a practitioner.

In countries like Australia, a growing number of private health insurance organisations provide cover, with some providing up to 70 per cent rebate for acupuncture and herbal therapies. However, this cover is currently only available to patients who have received treatment from members of TCM, acupuncture or natural therapies organisations recognised by these funds. A number of large government and private organisations also provide for TCM therapies in their health scheme.

Locating a good TCM practitioner

Being an aware consumer who knows what constitutes TCM, is helpful when trying to locate a good TCM practitioner in a country where registration does not exist. Exceptions are China, where TCM and Western medical practitioners are registered separately, and some American and Canadian States, where TCM practitioners are registered as acupuncturists or herbalists.

Inevitably, the level of training, skills and experience of TCM practitioners in states or countries varies where registration does not exist, so locating a good practitioner requires some initial investigation on the part of the consumer. Below is a checklist of useful considerations to guide the consumer.

Check the academic qualifications

A good TCM practitioner obviously must have a good, formal, higher-education qualification and some clinical training. This training should include TCM diagnostics, the main TCM disciplines and a degree of integrated training in Western medical disciplines, e.g. anatomy and physiology. Higher-education training in TCM or acupuncture may have been undertaken in China, Taiwan, Singapore, Korea or in countries in the West where TCM is taught in private educational institutions or in universities. Chinese medicine, acupuncture or natural therapy organisations may assist the consumer in finding out about the academic qualifications of a particular practitioner. These organisations can be found in metropolitan telephone directories. Perusal of displayed diplomas, degrees etc. in the practitioner's clinic is also advisable.

Check clinical experience

The skill of a TCM practitioner not only comes from academic training but, more importantly, from the progressive accumulation of clinical experience in diagnosing and treating various clinical conditions. In general terms, the longer the experience of a TCM practitioner, the more skilled he or she is.

The skills of a TCM practitioner can be measured in terms of the success achieved in dealing with various clinical conditions. Hence, the consumer is well advised to check either from friends or contacts as to the clinical reputation of a particular practitioner.

Check professional associations

As TCM gains acceptability in the West, codes of professional conduct will evolve in the practice of its various disciplines. In Australia, where acupuncture has gained a wider acceptability compared with other TCM disciplines, ethical and professional standards for its practice have been developed and propagated. The Acupuncture Ethics and Standards Organisation (AESO) has a comprehensive ethical and professional code for its members. These standards cover such areas as confidentiality of the patient, practitioner-patient relationships, relationships between acupuncture practitioners and other health professionals, patient records and publicity. Disciplinary actions such as the suspension or expulsion of a member may be instituted for professional misconduct.

In recent times various other TCM organisations in Australia have been working to draw up a unified code of ethics and professional standards to cover all the areas of TCM practice. Most TCM practitioners are members of TCM or acupuncture organisations. Some of these organisations have a referral service which directs consumers to the practitioner in their locality. If this service is available, check on the academic, professional and clinical skills of practitioners being referred.

Check linguistic and cross-cultural skills

TCM is a body of knowledge which was linguistically and culturally constructed in China. To apply and practise it successfully in a place with a different culture and linguistic medium means that the practitioner must not only possess the academic skills which give him or her access to this knowledge system but, more importantly, he or she must have the additional skills of being able to apply them flexibly in the new place. To successfully construct a clinical pattern of a particular patient in a Western setting, the practitioner must be able to speak the local language and understand the local culture and tradition. A TCM consumer therefore must look for good local linguistic skills and cross-cultural skills in a TCM practitioner.

• CHAPTER IV •

CHINESE HERBAL MEDICINE
中药

IN TRADITIONAL CHINESE MEDICINE, DISEASES MANIFEST THEMSELVES IN A multitude of clinical patterns. These clinical patterns, of which more than 2000 have been collated, observed and recorded, can indicate whether the disease is hot or cold in nature, located superficially or deep inside the body, developing acutely or slowly, and whether it is causing disharmony of the organ and channel systems.

In the long course of evolution, leaves, flowers, stems, roots and fruits of certain plants, as well as certain minerals and animal products, were found to redress defined clinical patterns. Initially, individual herbs were found to alleviate certain simple disease patterns. Subsequently, a combination of these and other substances were found to be efficacious in dealing with more complicated disease patterns.

By observing and experiencing the effects of herbs on several disease patterns, the medicinal and therapeutic attributes of 2300 individual and combined plant, animal and mineral substances were found and developed into 2900 formulae. Concurrently, a system of classification was devised which defined the 'nature' or 'character' and the therapeutic action of these herbs and substances vis-a-vis redressing the disharmony manifested in various clinical patterns.

Every medicinal substance therefore has a particular attribute, characteristic and therapeutic action which defines its main therapeutic or harmonising effect upon the body. This attribute, pian sheng 偏胜, is also termed 'inclination', 'deviation' or bias. Specifically, this means that every medicinal substance may be inclined towards being hot, cold, warm, cool, floating, sinking, moistening, drying, sweet, pungent, sour, salty, bitter, tonifying, sedating etc. In Chinese medical terms, it is the manipulation of these inclinations which brings about equilibrium or balance to a diseased clinical pattern or disharmony. In general terms, the fundamental principle in restoring harmony in Chinese medicine holds that 'when the pattern is hot, cool it; when cold, warm it; when deficient, tonify it; when excessive, purge it; when dry, moisten it; and when damp, dry it'.

1. THE FOUR QI ATTRIBUTES: HOT, COLD, WARM, COOL AND BLAND

Hot, cold, warm, cool and bland attributes, also referred to as Qi attributes, are the first set of basic criteria used to classify the therapeutic nature of Chinese herbs and other medicinal substances.

Herbs with hot or warm attributes (the difference being only one of degree) can be used for clinical patterns characterised by 'cold' symptoms, e.g. chills or lowered metabolic rate. Dried ginger and Japanese catnip are examples of hot and cold herbs respectively.

Conversely, herbs with cold or cooling attributes are used to balance clinical patterns characterised by heat or fevers. Examples of these herbs are mint leaves and stems, root of the Baical skullcap, honeysuckle flowers, forsythia fruits and bamboo leaves.

Finally, there also 'neutral' or ping herbs, which are neither hot, cold, warm nor cool. They may be used selectively in clinical patterns which require only slight balancing and where extremes of hot or warm and cold or cooling herbs might prove to be too strong. Examples of this category of herbs are licorice root and Chinese yam root or shan yao.

This method of classifying medicinal herbs was a product of many years of repeated observation structured by ancient philosophical thought. During the cold days of winter, for example, it was observed that after drinking boiled ginger tea, one feels warm throughout the body. Hence, it was concluded that ginger has a warm attribute. During the hot summer days, after eating watermelon, people experienced a cooling effect, hence the conclusion that watermelon has a cooling attribute.

This common experience extended to the eating of other substances and their application to more complicated clinical conditions. For example, in hot clinical patterns characterised by high fever, irritability and thirst, cold and cooling medicinal substances, such as gypsum and honeysuckle flowers were found to eliminate the heat. On the other hand, severe diarrhoea as a result of ingesting cold water or food — a cold clinical pattern — was found to be cured after the taking of herbs with a warming attribute, e.g. ginger.

THE FIVE HERB FLAVOURS

Pungent, sweet, sour, bitter and salty are the five flavours of individual medicinal substances. Any one substance may be classified under more than one type of flavour. In the unique evolution of herbal medicine in China, however, the five flavours have assumed meanings beyond their gustatory attributes. They have also all been differentiated and classified according to their characteristics and therapeutic qualities.

Pungent-flavoured herbs

Pungent-flavoured herbs generally taste tangy and have a dispersing inclination, which can enhance the opening of the skin pores and generate perspiration. For this reason they are commonly used for exterior patterns of disease where pathogenic Qi or factors of cold or heat may affect the exterior of the body. They also promote the flow of Qi along the acupuncture channels.

Typical examples of pungent-flavoured herbs are ginger, perilla leaves, forsythia fruit, Japanese catnip, mandarin peel and root of the balloon flower.

Sweet-flavoured herbs

Sweet-flavoured herbs, which are not always sweet to taste, have tonifying, moistening, relaxing and soothing inclinations. Hence, they are generally used for deficient clinical patterns. Examples include ginseng, licorice root, bamboo leaves, honeysuckle and honey.

Sour-flavoured herbs

Sour-flavoured herbs generally have a 'gathering' and astringent effect and so are commonly used for deficient clinical patterns with symptoms of profuse sweating, diarrhoea or seminal emission. These conditions are brought about by Qi deficiency, resulting in the body's inability to hold back secretions of vital fluids. Examples of these substances are Schizandra fruit, oyster shells, hawthorn fruit.

Bitter-flavoured herbs

Bitter-flavoured herbs, which generally have the inclination to dry dampness and clear or move pathogenic heat or fire downwards, are commonly used for damp and hot patterns and those reflecting obstruction of the Qi and blood. They are usually administered to patients suffering from high fevers, such as in influenza or pneumonia. They facilitate the elimination of dampness and mucus in the body and also remove obstructions in the bowel, blood vessels and acupuncture channels. Examples of bitter-flavoured herbs are prepared soya bean, golden thread, rhubarb root, cork tree bark and atractolydis root.

Salty-flavoured herbs

Salty-flavoured herbs have the inclination to soften hard, accumulated mass, promote the downward movement of the Qi and thus act as a purgative. They are used for clinical patterns involving abnormal tissue growth like goiters, tumours, lymph node inflammation, as well as for accumulated faeces within the bowel in cases of constipation. Examples of these medicinal substances are abalone shells, oyster shells and mirabilite.

A comparative study done in China on the percentage of convergence of the categorisation of the flavour of about 64 different types of herbs and their *actual* taste or flavour revealed a 43.5 per cent convergence.

As for the chemical composition of herbs with pungent, bitter, sweet, sour and salty herbs, a separate study shows that most pungent herbs contain volatile oils; bitter-tasting herbs mainly contain alkaloids and glucosides; sweet-flavoured herbs mainly contain nutrients such as amino acid and sugar; sour-tasting herbs mainly contain tannin and organic acids; while salty herbs mainly contain organic salt, sodium sulphate and iodine.

FOUR DIRECTIONS *Si Xiang* 四向

Depending upon their texture, mass, lightness or heaviness, medicinal substances may be classified into ascending, floating, descending or sinking herbs.

Substances with ascending or floating inclinations are light in weight and mass, e.g. flowers and leaves, and have the general effect of lifting the Qi, counteracting cold pathogenic factors and dispelling disease factors on the exterior of the body. Examples are the magnolia flower and the lotus leaf.

On the other hand, substances with descending or sinking inclinations, e.g. (mostly seeds and fruits) promote a downward and inward motion and have the generalised effect of checking an over-active yang Qi and bringing down a rising pathogenic Qi in conditions with symptoms of vomiting, fever, dizziness etc. They also have an astringent effect in that they bring down heat and fever, promote movement of the body fluids, act as diuretics and facilitate bowel motion. Examples of the descending and sinking herbs are perilla seeds, prepared rhizome of *Rehmannia glutinosa* (shu di) and magnetite (ci shi).

Medicinal substances with pungent and sweet flavours as well as hot and warm attributes mostly bring about ascending or floating actions. Examples are the ephedra and cassia twigs. These have a generalised yang effect. Substances with bitter, sour and salty flavours and a cold attribute usually have a descending or sinking action. This may be generalised as a yin inclination. Examples are mirabilite (meng xiao), Chinese peony (shao yao) and oyster shells (mu li).

Preparation and processing of raw herbs or pao zhi also affects the inclination of herbs. When herbs are stir-fried with spirits or wine, this will boost their ascending and floating effect; with ginger juice, their dispersing effect; with vinegar, their gathering effect; and with salt, their descending or sinking inclination. When ascending and floating herbs are combined with a greater number of descending or sinking herbs, a descending or sinking effect will tend to be the outcome. On the other hand, when descending or sinking herbs are combined with a greater number of ascending or floating herbs it will tend to produce an upward floating effect.

ACUPUNCTURE CHANNEL ATTRIBUTE *Gui Jing* 归经

Substances are given specific organ(s) and channel-systems attributes if they are effective in treating a disharmony in the same. Specifically, their attributes are linked with one or more organ systems, i.e. the heart, liver, kidneys, spleen, lungs, stomach, small and large intestines, gall bladder, triple energiser (see glossary) and pericardium; and the twelve acupuncture channels which relate to these organ systems.

The use of such attributes can be clearly illustrated in the herbal treatment of headaches. In TCM headaches may be differentiated into various clinical patterns depending upon the patient's perceived site of pain. Site can indicate particular channel disharmonies. A back-of-the-head headache which extends to the neck is a sign of disharmony of the greater yang channel, which connects with the urinary bladder and small intestine systems. For this pattern of headache, the herb *Rhizoma notoptergyii* (qiang huo) which has a urinary bladder channel attribute, is used.

A headache on the forehead extending to the eyebrows indicates diseases affecting the bright yang channel, which connects with the stomach and large intestine systems. For this clinical pattern, the herb *Radix angelica* (bai zhi), classified under the stomach channel attribute, is found to be effective.

A headache on both sides of the head indicates disharmony of the lesser yang channel which connects with the gall bladder and triple energiser systems. The root of Sichuan lovage (chuan xiong), classified under the gall bladder channel attribute, is effective for this condition.

A top-of-the-head headache extending to the eyes indicates a disease pattern of the terminal yin channel which connects with the liver and pericardium systems. This pattern is treated with Evodia fruit (wu zhu yu) which is categorised as having a liver channel attribute.

As for an example of a herb classified under an organ system, we can cite the example of the apricot kernel (xing ren) which has been confirmed by repeated use to stop coughing and asthmatic wheezing, symptoms which are associated with disharmony of the lung system. Hence, apricot kernel is classified as having a lung system attribute. Clinical patterns involving pain, itchiness and sores are reflections of diseases implicating the heart system. Hence, herbs found to be effective against these disease patterns are grouped under the heart system attribute .

THERAPEUTIC ACTION *Gong Xiao* OF HERBS

The four Qi attributes, the five flavours, the four directions and the acupuncture channel attributes form a 'four-in-one' combination which constitutes the foundation for determining and delineating the therapeutic action gong xiao of herbs and other medicinal substances. Below are the major general categories of therapeutic action under which thousands of substances are subdivided. This English-language system of categorisation was patterned after Bensky's table of contents in his book *Chinese Herbal Medicine, Materia Medica*. Substances in these groups can:

1. Release exterior patterns
2. Clear heat patterns
3. Drain downwards
4. Dry dampness
5. Expel wind dampness
6. Transform phlegm and stop coughing
7. Transform dampness

8. Relieve food stagnation
9. Regulate the Qi
10. Regulate the blood
11. Warm the interior and expel cold pathogens
12. Tonify
13. Act as an astringent
14. Calm the spirit
15. Open the orifices
16. Extinguish wind and stop tremors
17. Expel parasites

Some commonly used Chinese Herbs

Ginseng Root *Panax ginseng* Ren Shen 人参

Qi Attribute:	Slightly warm
Flavour:	Sweet, slightly bitter
Channel Attribute:	Spleen and lungs
Therapeutic Action:	Tonifies original Qi and lungs and spleen systems

'Ren' refers to a person, while 'shen' refers to the constellation Orion or is a pun on another word 'shen' 神 , which means spirit or magical. The shape of the ginseng root is similar to that of a human form, hence the name 'ren'. Ginseng is most often used as a medicine of last resort for critical life and death clinical conditions. Hence, ginseng is referred to in Chinese as 'shen cao' or magical herb.

Ginseng root has a sweet and slightly warm Qi, so it is commonly used as a tonifying agent, being a major tonic for the body's original Qi. Original Qi is the vital energy from which all other Qi comes. Once this Qi has been depleted (as a result of prolonged illness, loss of blood, severe diarrhoea or profuse sweating) the Qi deficiency may be so severe that the condition becomes critical. This clinical pattern falls within the scope of the therapeutic action of ginseng root. Ginseng root may also be used to deal with clinical patterns involving spleen or lung organ deficiency.

There are two main types of ginseng, the very expensive wild species called the 'wild mountain root' or ye shan shen, which grows in the north-west regions of China and in Korea; and the relatively inexpensive varieties, i.e. 'white root ginseng', 'dried root ginseng' and the American ginseng (*Panacis quinquefolii*).

Five to ten grams of ginseng root is boiled with water using moderate heat and administered orally by itself or mixed with a decoction made from other herbs. In critical cases, this dosage may be increased to 15–20 grams with the decoction administered orally in portions. Ginseng may also be powdered and administered in the dosage of 0.5–1 gram orally, twice a day.

Due to the slightly warm attribute and sweet flavour of this herb, it is not used for conditions with heat patterns; or signs and symptoms of hypertension. (Heat patterns require sedation, not tonification with the use of sweet and warm herbs.)

Dang Gui Root *Angelica sinensis* Dang Gui 当归

Qi Attribute:	Warm
Flavour:	Pungent, bitter, sweet
Channel Attribute:	Heart, liver, spleen
Therapeutic Action:	Tonifies blood, enlivens blood flow and stops pain

While ginseng root is a Qi tonic, Dang Gui root is a blood tonic. It is thus used for a blood deficiency clinical pattern with symptoms of fatigue, dizziness, pale yellow facial complexion and very pale lips and fingernails as commonly seen in anaemic patients. This pungent-flavoured herb is also very commonly used for menstrual complaints, e.g. period pains and irregular periods because it can enliven blood circulation and stop pain. In addition, it can also moisten the intestines and alleviate constipation caused by prolonged illness, physical debility or blood deficiency after childbirth.

The dosage is 5–15 grams, which may be combined and decocted with other herbs. It may also be soaked in spirits for a period of time, after which the spirit is taken orally.

Because of its sweet flavour and inclination to moisten the intestines, caution is required for patients with diarhoea. It is not advisable for patients with yin deficiency patterns and signs of heat.

Peppermint *Mentha arvensis* Bo He 薄荷

Qi Attribute:	Cooling
Flavour:	Pungent and aromatic
Channel Attribute:	Lung and liver
Therapeutic Action:	Disperses pathogenic wind and heat, benefits the throat and eliminates liver system Qi stagnation

Peppermint or mint leaves are herbs commonly used for releasing exterior heat patterns with symptoms of fever, no perspiration, slight aversion to wind or cold, headache and pain all over the body, in fact the symptoms of the common cold.

Due to its liver channel attribute and pungent flavour, peppermint can promote the flow of liver Qi. It can thus deal with a constrained flow of liver Qi which manifests itself in clinical patterns with symptoms of congestion in the chest and flanks accompanied by some emotional depression.

The dosage is 2–10 grams. It is not advisable to boil this herb for too long, but rather add it after boiling the other herbs in a formula.

This herb is not advisable for patients suffering from severe sweating due to a deficient clinical pattern; and a hyperactive liver yang.

Tangerine Peel *Citrus reticulata blanco* Chen Pi 陈皮

Qi Attribute:	Warm
Flavour:	Pungent and bitter
Channel Attribute:	Spleen, stomach, lungs
Therapeutic Action:	Regulates Qi flow, dries dampness and transforms phlegm

This is the dried and sliced peel of a ripened orange, mandarin or tangerine. It is one of the major Qi flow regulators. Specifically, it regulates the Qi flow of the stomach and spleen system and is used to deal with clinical patterns involving Qi stagnation of these organ systems. This clinical pattern manifests symptoms of indigestion, abdominal distention, loss of appetite, nausea or vomiting.

For a slight condition displaying this clinical pattern, 10 grams of tangerine peel is mixed with boiling water and then taken orally like tea.

Because of its warm Qi and lung channel attributes, peel can dry dampness and disperse phlegm affecting the lung system. It is thus used to treat the clinical patterns of coughing with substantial white-coloured phlegm expectoration accompanied by chest congestion.

Normal dosage is 3–9 grams. Due to its pungent, bitter flavour and warm Qi attribute, peel can generate heat in the body. Hence caution must be observed when prescribing it for patients with internal heat manifested in a clinical pattern of a red tongue with little moisture. It is not advisable for patients with a Qi or yin deficient clinical pattern, or an unproductive dry cough.

Cinnamon Twigs *Cinnamomum cassia* Gui Zhi 桂枝

Qi Attribute:	Warm
Flavour:	Pungent, sweet
Channel Attribute:	Lung, urinary bladder
Therapeutic Action:	Dispels wind-cold exterior pattern, promotes yang Qi flow along the channels

While peppermint is used to deal with exterior heat patterns, cinnamon twigs, due to their warm Qi attribute, pungent flavour and lung channel attribute, are used to deal with exterior cold patterns. Exterior cold patterns, which are generally found in the initial stages of a flu or cold, exhibit symptoms of chills and aversion to cold or wind while fever symptoms are not very marked.

Due to their warm attributes cinnamon twigs can also warm the channels and disperse cold pathogenic factors, thereby making them suitable for joint and period pains.

Cinnamon twigs may be decocted with other herbs or used as an ingredient in herb tablets. Dosage is 5–10 grams.

Due to their warm Qi attribute, these herbs are not advisable for patterns of yin deficiency with signs of heat or warm-febrile diseases in which patterns of symptoms and signs may include those of infectious viral and bacterial diseases.

Licorice Root *Glycyrrhiza uralensis* Gan Cao 甘草

Qi Attribute:	Neutral (raw), warm (toasted)
Flavour:	Sweet
Channel Attribute:	All primary 12 channels (mainly spleen and lung systems)
Therapeutic Action:	Tonifies deficient spleen system, moistens the lung system and stops coughing, soothes, relieves and stops pain

The literal translation of this herb is 'sweet herb'. Its neutral Qi and 12 primary channel attributes makes it highly valued by Chinese herbalists because of its harmonising and correcting effect when combined with other herbs.

Due to its sweet flavour and channel attribute, which centres on the spleen organ system, licorice root can tonify the spleen Qi and address a spleen Qi deficiency pattern characterised by symptoms of weakness, shortness of breath and a weak pulse.

It has an inclination to soothe and relax spasms and pain conditions (especially in the abdomen and extremities) due to its sweet flavour inclination. Raw licorice root also has a detoxifying effect and so it is used for treating different forms of poisoning.

For internal administration, the dosage is 3–10 grams. Prolonged oral administration of this herb in large doses, however, can bring about symptoms of tissue fluid retention, hypertension, weakness, shaking in the extremities, dizziness and headaches due to electrolytic imbalance involving sodium and potassium.

It is not advisable for patterns with a preponderance of damp characterised by symptoms of chest and abdominal congestion or for vomiting. This is because its sweet attribute can build up dampness and Qi congestion within the chest and abdomen.

Gypsum *Calcium sulphate* Shi Gao 石膏

Qi Attribute:	Very cold
Flavour:	Sweet and pungent
Channel Attribute:	Lungs and stomach
Therapeutic Action:	Brings down heat and fire; stops thirst

Gypsum is a mineral substance of which the main chemical content is calcium sulphate. Only the soft, not the hard type of gypsum is used for herbal medicine. Medicinal gypsum can be taken in the raw (sheng shi gao) or baked (duan shi gao) forms depending on the therapeutic action required.

Raw gypsum, which has a very cold Qi attribute, is very effective for heat draining (its heavy weight and texture gives it a strong sinking and descending inclination). It is thus very commonly used for disease patterns exhibiting symptoms of high fever.

In addition, raw gypsum is used to clear heat from the stomach system which manifests itself in stomach fire disease patterns with symptoms of headache, toothache or swollen and painful gums. Raw gypsum's very cold attribute and heat draining capacity enables it to be used to clear heat from the lung system and thus indirectly to stop coughing.

When used as an ingredient in a herbal decoction, it is boiled ahead of the other herbs. The dosage is usually quite high, from 15–60 grams. It is not advised for weak stomachs and deficient yang clinical patterns.

Baked gypsum is commonly used externally in powdered form to clear skin heat patterns with symptoms of eczema, ulcerated sores, etc.

Velvet Deer Antlers Lu Rong 鹿茸

Qi Attribute:	Warm
Flavour:	Sweet-salty
Channel Attribute:	Liver, kidneys
Therapeutic Action:	Tonifies kidney yang, constitutional essence and blood, strengthens tendons and bones

This medicinal substance is made from the velvet of two species of male deer: *Cervis nippon* and the red deer *Cervis elaphus*.

The antler can either be cleaned and powdered or processed in a particular way and then cut into thin slices ready for use. The deers suffer no ill-effect in losing their antlers.

Being sweet in Qi attribute, the deer antler is a tonifying agent. It primarily tonifies the yang Qi and, since its channel attribute is the kidney channel, it is mainly used to tonify a deficient kidney yang. A deficient kidney yang pattern includes symptoms of impotence, coldness in the extremities (especially the feet) and lack of strength in the lower back and lower extremities. Antlers can also strengthen the bones and sinews, and bolster healing in bone fractures.

In women, a deficient yang Qi can manifest itself in patterns with symptoms of excessive vaginal emission, excessive and continuous menstrual bleeding and infertility. For this clinical pattern, deer antler alone is administered.

The dosage for the oral administration is 1–2 grams which may be taken in powdered form or mixed with other herbs and decocted. A small dosage can have an excitory effect, while a large dose can increase libido.

It is not advised for patterns of yin deficiency with signs of heat, due to the fact that its warm Qi attribute can boost the yang Qi in the body.

Honeysuckle Flower *Lonicera japonica* Jin Yin Hua 金银花

Qi Attribute:	Cold
Flavour:	Sweet
Channel Attribute:	Lung, stomach
Therapeutic Action:	Clears heat and detoxifies

Honeysuckle has a cold attribute and, being a flower which is light in weight, has a floating and ascending inclination. Therefore it is used to clear heat, especially in wind-heat exterior patterns, heat patterns manifesting themselves as skin sores, swellings or abcesses along the exterior of the body and warm febrile diseases. For the pattern of damp-heat diarrhoea it is used with other herbs but if the pattern includes some bleeding, it is stir-fried until black. Dosage is 10–20 grams.

Sour Date Seed *Ziziphus jujuba* var. *spinosa* Suan Zao Ren 酸枣仁

Qi Attribute:	Neutral
Flavour:	Sour, sweet
Channel Attribute:	Heart, spleen, liver, gall bladder
Therapeutic Action:	Nourishes heart system, calms the spirit, holds back sweat

Sour date seed is typical of the herbs which calm the spirit. If the blood is deficient, the heart loses its nourishment and cannot 'house the spirit'. Under this situation, disease patterns of heart fire emerge, characterised by symptoms of irritability, insomnia, palpitations and anxiety. The sweet flavour, neutral Qi attribute and heavy texture of the sour date bring about a therapeutic action. The 'gathering' or astringent inclination from its sour flavour makes it suitable for treating night sweats and spontaneous sweating brought on by organ system deficiency.

The seeds are pounded into pieces before use. When used raw, they address deficient patterns with signs of heat. When the seeds are stir-fried the attribute transforms from a neutral to a warm Qi which in turn strengthens its tonifying qualities. Dosage: 10–18 grams.

HERB FORMULAE *Fang Ji* 方剂

The art of composing a herb formula to fit a particular clinical pattern has evolved in China over several thousand years. It is the knowledge of each herb's 'inclination' which determines with which other herbs it should be combined to fit a particular clinical pattern. In some cases, where a clinical pattern presents itself clearly, the choice of herbs will be easy. For example, in cases of heat pathogenic factors affecting the lung organ system with symptoms of cough, fever, reddish tongue and rapid pulse, the practitioner would choose cooling herbs which have lung channel attributes.

However, in most cases clinical patterns are very complicated. They can involve a merging of hot and cold, deficient and excess, external and internal patterns, etc. Under these conditions, knowledge and experience is needed.

On the basis of long practice and observation, it was discovered that combining individual herbs with their individual inclinations brought about clinical changes. Some individual herbs or a group of herbs can increase or decrease the therapeutic efficacy of another herb; some can enhance or decrease the toxic effect or side effects of others, and so on. From repeated experience, a body of knowledge, referred to as the 'seven conditions', qi qing 七情, has developed into a system of safe, therapeutic and efficacious herbal prescriptions.

The seven conditions in herb combination

1. **Single herb or dan xing**: an example of this is the use of ginseng (du shen tang) to tonify the Qi.

2. **Reinforcing or xiang xu**: the combination of more than two different herbs with similar therapeutic efficacy or inclinations to mutually enhance their therapeutic effects. For example, a combination of the root of *Anemarrhenae asphodeloidis* (zhi mu) and cork tree bark (huang bai) enhances both herbs' common efficacy of nourishing the yin and bringing down the fire.

3. **Complementary or xiang shi**: when two herbs, a major and an auxiliary one, are combined so that the auxiliary herb enhances the therapeutic effect of the major herb. In the combination of milk-vetch root (huang qi) and China root (fu ling), the latter enhances milk-vetch root's Qi tonifying and diuretic effects.

4. **Restraining or xiang wei**: when one herb is used to restrain the strong inclination or toxic effect of another, e.g. fresh ginger is used with *Pinellia ternata* (ban xia) to restrain the latter's toxicity.

5. **Counteracting or xiang sha:** the use of one herb to eliminate another's toxicity e.g. mung bean is used to counteract poisoning from *Croton tiglium* (ba dou).

6. **Supression or xiang e**: the use of one herb to nullify the efficacy of another, e.g. radish seeds (lai fu zi) are prohibited from being used together with ginseng as it would nullify ginseng's Qi tonifying therapeutic effect.

7. **Side-effects or xiang fan**: the combination of two herbs to produce negative side-effects, e.g. licorice root (gan cao) is prohibited from being com-

bined with *Euphorbia kansui* (gan sui) as it would produce side-effects.

Of all the above methods of combining herbs, the reinforcing and complementary are the most commonly used. Restraining and counteracting methods are commonly used for herbs with toxic effects, while the supression and side-effects methods fall under the category of prohibited herb combinations because the desired therapeutic action will not be achieved and severe or fatal side-effects could result.

Composing a Chinese herbal prescription

A common herbal formula can contain more than 12 different individual herbs, which are listed together with instructions for the method of preparation, administration and dosage. The herbalist signs and dates the written formula. Every compound herbal formula has four main components which are named and written in a prescription like the line-up of royalties in a chess game:

1. **Principal ingredient.** This herb or combination of herbs provides the main therapeutic thrust of the prescription since it deals with the main signs or symptoms of a clinical pattern. The names of these herbs are normally written at the head of the list in the prescription. Since they play a decisive role in dealing with the 'enemy' (the clinical pattern), they are referred to as the 'king' (jun).

2. **Adjuvant or complementary ingredients.** This group of herbs complements the action of the principal ingredients, so they are referred to as 'ministers' or officials under the monarch (chen). They may be equivalent to the queen in the game of chess.

3. **Correctant ingredients.** This group of herbal ingredients tempers the action of the principal ingredient or relieves secondary symptoms. They are referred to as the 'court official' (zuo) and are equivalent to the bishop in chess.

4. **Actant ingredients.** These are the herbal ingredients which direct the therapeutic effects towards the relevant channel or site. They supposedly implement the decisions of the monarch and act on them; hence the name 'royal envoy' (shi). They may be compared with the pawns in chess.

These actants have a guiding influence among the other ingredients in the prescription in the sense that they can change the channel attribute of other ingredients and concentrate the main therapeutic thrust of the prescription towards the channel site of the illness.

Some designated actants are classified in accordance with their channel attributes. For example, the main actant for the stomach channel is gypsum and for the kidney channel, it is cinnamon bark.

Below is a dissection of a Qing-dynasty (1644–1911) herbal prescription which is a common prescription still used by TCM practitioners to deal with the external wind-heat clinical pattern. This prescription is named 'honeysuckle forsythia combination' or yin qiao san 银翘散.

Principal ingredients

Honeysuckle flower (cold/sweet)	30 grams
Forsythia fruit (cool/pungent/bitter)	30 grams

Adjuvants

Peppermint (cool/pungent)	18 grams
Prepared soya beans (neutral/bitter/sweet)	15 grams
Bamboo leaves (cold/sweet)	12 grams

Correctants

Japanese catnip (warm/pungent)	12 grams
Balloon flower root (neutral/bitter)	18 grams
Great burdock fruit (cool/bitter/pungent)	18 grams

Actant

Licorice root (neutral/sweet)	15 grams

(The weights given are so high because they were to be powdered and taken over several days. A decoction would be one-fifth of these weights.)

The signs and symptoms of an external wind-heat clinical pattern are: fever, slight aversion to cold or wind, no sweating or spasmodic sweating, headache, thirst, cough, sore throat, redness on tip of tongue, thin white tongue coat, and a rapid and superficial pulse.

The main ingredients, honeysuckle flower and forsythia fruit, have a predominantly cold Qi attribute with sweet and bitter flavours. They are used to disperse the pathogenic heat and wind affecting the exterior, characterised by symptoms of fever, slight aversion to wind or cold, redness on the tip of the tongue and rapid pulse.

The adjuvants, peppermint, prepared soya beans and Japanese catnip, have predominantly cold and cool Qi attributes and pungent flavours which chiefly enhance the efficacy of the main ingredients. Japanese catnip, which has a warm Qi attribute, balances the predominantly cold nature of the prescription, thus acting as a correctant. The other correctants (root of balloon flower and great burdock fruit) deal with the secondary symptoms of cough and sore throat. Licorice root plays the role of the actant which harmonises all the ingredients.

COMMON HERB FORMULAE

Below are examples of herb formulae classifed in accordance with the herbal ingredient's system of organisation.

Mulberry and Chrysanthemum Combination or San Ju Yin 桑菊饮

1. Mulberry leaf (sang ye 桑叶)	8 grams
2. Chrysanthemum flower (ju hua 菊花)	6 grams
3. Apricot kernel (xing ren 杏仁)	6 grams
4. Root of balloon flower (jie gang 桔更)	6 grams
5. Licorice root (gan cao 甘草)	2 grams
6. Peppermint (bo he 薄荷) (mixed after boiling)	6 grams
7. Forsythia fruit (lian qiao 连翘)	6 grams
8. Reed rhizome (lu gen 芦根)	6 grams

Mulberry and chrysanthemum combination is considered a small prescription or xiao fang in the sense that it uses few ingredients in small doses to deal with a slight disease pattern. This prescription is used to deal with the initial stage of a wind-heat pathogenic attack on the exterior, the main signs and symptoms of which are fever, slight aversion to cold or wind, cough, thirst etc.

In this formula, the primary herbal ingredients, the mulberry leaf and the chrysanthemum flower, are both sweet-flavoured herbs with cool Qi attributes while having lung channel attributes. Together, they can clear the wind-heat from the exterior. Peppermint, which has a cool Qi attribute and pungent flavour, can assist the above ingredients in dispelling wind-heat. Apricot kernel, having a heavy texture with descending inclinations, can bring down the lung Qi; while the fruit of the balloon flower spreads the lung Qi. The combination of the descending and spreading inclinations can restore the lung system's ventilating functions and thus stop coughing. Peppermint, apricot kernel and the fruit of the balloon flower are all adjuvants.

Forsythia fruit, with its cold Qi attribute, pungent flavour and a light texture, can penetrate the exterior and clear the heat. Reed rhizome, with a cold Qi attribute and sweet flavour, clears the heat and enhances body fluid production, thus alleviating thirst. Both are correctants. Licorice is the actant in this prescription.

Four Major Herbs Combination or Si Jun Zi Tang 四君子汤

1. Ginseng (ren shen 人参)	12 grams
2. *Rhizoma atractylodis* (bai zhu 白术)	9 grams
3. China root (fu ling 茯苓)	9 grams
4. Licorice root (gan cao 甘草) (toasted)	5 grams

Four Major Herbs Combination is a moderating formula or huan fang. This type of formula is administered for a protracted period of time and has a gradual therapeutic effect on chronic debilitating illnesses. It is used to deal with a spleen and stomach Qi deficiency, the signs and symptoms of which are a loss of appetite, nausea, loose bowel motions or diarrhoea, abdominal sounds, lack of strength in the four extremities, a pale facial complexion, a low-pitched voice, pale tongue body with a thin white tongue coating and a weak and empty pulse.

In this formula, ginseng is the primary herb ingredient. It gives great tonification to the spleen and stomach Qi. Once the spleen and stomach Qi are tonified, the spleen and stomach function of transforming essence from food will be restored and symptoms of loss of appetite, lack of strength in the extremities and weak pulse will be addressed.

Rhizoma atractylodis, with a warm Qi attribute and bitter flavour, can dry dampness created by a weak spleen and stomach Qi and thus alleviate symptoms of diarrhoea. China root can promote the passing of excessive dampness through urination. These two have a mutually reinforcing effect. Toasted licorice, with a warm Qi attribute and a sweet flavour, can tonify the spleen and stomach Qi.

Four Cold Limbs Combination Si Ni Tang 四逆汤

1. Prepared Sichuan aconite (fu zi 附子)   9 grams
   (Aconite is a scheduled substance in Australia and its use is restricted to doctors, dentists and vets.)
2. Dried ginger (gan jiang 干姜)   9 grams
3. Licorice root (gan cao 甘草) (toasted)   12 grams

Four Cold Limbs Combination is an 'emergency formula' or ji fang. Emergency prescriptions use herb ingredients which have strong inclination to deal with critical disease patterns that require urgent treatment or achieve rapid recovery. This formula is used for a yang exhaustion disease pattern, the signs and symptoms of which are cold limbs, aversion to cold with a curled body, vomiting, abdominal pains, watery diarrhoea with undigested food, tiredness and sleepiness, no thirst, a pale tongue body with a smooth and white tongue coating and a deep and thin pulse.

In this formula, prepared Sichuan aconite, which has a very hot Qi attribute and a very pungent flavour, is used as the principal ingredient to tonify the kidney yang, dispel pathogenic cold and revive the patient from a critical condition. Dried ginger, with a warm Qi attribute, assists the prepared Sichuan aconite to restore the depleted yang. In this prescription, licorice is used as an actant. It can simultaneously regulate all the ingredients in the prescription and counteract the extreme heat and pungent flavour generated by the prepared aconite and dried ginger. In addition, licorice and dried ginger can warm the spleen yang.

Poria Five Combination or Wu Ling San 五苓散

1. Water plantain (ze xie 泽泻)   15 grams
2. Poria (fu ling 茯苓)   9 grams
3. *Polyporus umbellatus* (zhu ling 猪苓)   9 grams
4. *Rhizoma atractylodis* (bai zhu 白术)   9 grams
5. Cinnamon twigs (gui zhi 桂枝)   6 grams

Poria Five Combination is considered an 'odd-number' herbal formula. All single and odd-number ingredients in formulae are categorised as odd-number herb formulae. This type of herbal ingredient organisation is used to treat a recent illness which is not very severe or deep-seated. Odd-number formulae are categorised as yang arrangements, suited to counteract yin conditions.

The above herbal formula of five ingredients deals with a clinical pattern in which there is an exterior pathogen pattern, as well as stagnation of body fluids and internal dampness. The main signs and symptoms of this pattern are: headache and fever, thirst and desire to drink fluids, vomiting after fluid intake, difficulty in urination, a white coating of the tongue and a superficial pulse. This is a condition in which an exterior clinical pattern has not been dealt with effectively and has moved internally, specifically into the urinary bladder system. The main thrust of the treatment should be to facilitate urination and release the exterior pathogen.

In the prescription Poria Five Combination, water plantain, which has both neutral Qi and cold attributes, can promote urination and deal with the heat pathogen respectively. This is the primary ingredient. The other herb, poria, which has a neutral Qi attribute, can aid urination and hence reinforce the water plantain's effects. At the same time poria's warm Qi attribute boosts the yang Qi of the body to dispel dampness. *Polyporus umbellatus* has a bitter flavour which can unblock stagnation and a warm Qi attribute which can boost the yang Qi and neutral Qi attribute, to also promote urination. Hence these two herbs are the adjuvants in this prescription.

Rhizoma atractylodis has a warm Qi attribute and a sweet flavour. Its sweet flavour can tonify the spleen Qi which can boost the latter's capacity to move stagnant fluid. Cinnamon twig is the actant in this prescription. Its warm Qi attribute can warm the urinary bladder system to promote urination, and its pungent flavour can dispel any exterior pathogen.

Four Herbs Combination or Si Wu Tang 四物汤

1. Dangui root (dang gui 当归)   10 grams
2. Sichuan lovage root (chuan xiong 川芎)   6 grams
3. Peony root (bai shao 白芍)   10 grams
4. *Rehmannia glutinosa* (shou di 熟地) (toasted in wine)   15 grams

This is an even-number herbal combination. This type of organisation of herb ingredients is suitable for chronic, serious and deep-seated ailments.

Four Herbs Combination is commonly used to deal with a blood deficiency and blood stasis disease pattern, the signs and symptoms of which are dizziness, a proneness to fright, tinnitus, no lustre in the fingernails, a scanty or ceased menstrual period, pain along the navel, a pale tongue body; and a taut, thin pulse.

In this prescription, the principal herbs are the *Rehmannia glutinosa* and peony root. Both nourish the blood in the liver organ system and thus promote its function of storing blood. Dangui root is a common gynaecological herb. Its warm Qi attribute and pungent flavour promote the flow of Qi along the channels to stop pain and to tonify and enliven the blood flow. The Sichuan lovage root, with its warm Qi attribute and pungent flavour, reinforces the dangui root's capacity to promote Qi, blood circulation and to stop pain.

White Tiger Combination or Bai Hu Tang 白虎汤

1. Gypsum (shi gao 石膏)   30 grams
2. *Anemarrhena asphodeloides* (zhi mu 知母)   9 grams
3. Licorice root (gan cao 甘草) (toasted)   3 grams
4. Rice (jing mi 粳米)   9 grams

White Tiger Combination is a prescription which is suitable for the clinical pattern of pathogenic heat attacking the Qi layer of the body. This includes signs and symptoms of a very high fever, headache, a dry mouth and tongue, thirst and drinking, a flushed face and aversion to heat, profuse sweating and a big and strong or slippery but rapid pulse.

The primary ingredient in this prescription is gypsum. Its very cold Qi attribute and pungent flavour can dispel heat from the Qi layer of the body, pushing it towards the exterior and enhancing the production of body fluids to stop thirst. Its stomach and lung channel attributes enable it to clear heat in these organ systems.

Anemarrhena, the adjuvant, while having a bitter flavour and a cold Qi attribute, has a moistening nature and thus can clear heat from the stomach and lung Qi, thus reinforcing gypsum's heat-clearing effects. Licorice and rice can regulate the stomach function and conserve the body fluids while moderating the very cold Qi attribute and heavy descending nature of gypsum and *Anemarrhena*. They can also enhance by 'directing' the other herbs' effects on the stomach system, hence their role as actants.

Rehmannia Six Combination or Liu Wei Di Huang Wan 六味地黄丸

1. *Rehmannia glutinosa* (di huang 地黄)   24 grams
2. Chinese yam root (shan yao 山药)   12 grams
3. Asian Cornelian cherry fruit (shan yu rou 山萸肉)   12 grams
4. Water plantain (ze xie 泽泻)   9 grams
5. Poria (fu ling 茯苓)   9 grams
6. Cortex of tree peony root (mu dan pi 牡丹皮)   9 grams

Rehmannia Six Combination is a formula used to deal with kidney yin deficiency pattern, the signs and symptoms of which are lower back soreness, dizziness, tinnitus, hearing difficulties, night sweats, seminal emissions, regularly recurring fever, heat on the soles and palms, loosening of the teeth, a red tongue body and a deep, thin and rapid pulse. In this prescription a combination of three herbs tonify and another three herbs purge or sedate.

Foxglove root, the principal ingredient, is used to tonify the kidney yin. The Asian Cornelian cherry fruit with its sour flavour is used to gather and strengthen the yin and thus assist the foxglove root in tonifying the kidney yin. The poria is used to tonify the spleen yin system. So the three herbs form a 'troika' to tonify the body's yin.

Generally, internal heat emerges in cases of kidney yin deficiency, so water plantain is used to purge heat from the kidneys. The cortex of tree peony root is used to purge the liver heat.

Sour Date Seed Combination or Suan Zao Ren Tang 酸枣仁汤

1. Sour date seed (suan zao ren 酸枣仁)   18 grams
2. Poria (fu ling 茯苓)   6 grams
3. *Anemarrhena asphodeloides* (zhi mu 知母)   6 grams
4. Sichuan lovage root (chuan xiong 川芎)   3 grams
5. Licorice root (gan cao 甘草)   3 grams

Sour Date Seed Combination is a common formula used for a particular type of insomnia. It is a clinical pattern due to deficiency of the liver blood, the signs and symptoms of which are restlessness, failure to sleep, palpitations, night sweats, dizziness, a dry throat and mouth and a taut or thin and rapid pulse.

In this formula, sour date seed, with neutral Qi and liver channel attributes and a sour and sweet flavour, is the primary ingredient. Its sweet flavour can nourish the blood and settle the heart, while its sour flavour and neutral Qi attribute can gather the yin and stop the night sweats. The Sichuan lovage root's warm Qi attribute and pungent flavour can facilitate Qi movement, which subsequently enlivens blood flow and so enhances the free flow of the liver Qi. Poria can tonify the spleen and settle the heart. This assists the sour date seeds' action of settling the heart and spirit. The herb *Anemarrhena asphodeloides* can nourish the yin and move the heat downwards, moisten dryness and thus eliminate restlessness. The sweet flavour of licorice root is used to moderate the uneasiness of the liver.

Eight Precious Herbs Combination or Ba Zhen Tang 八珍汤

This is an example of what is referred to as a 'compound formula' or fu fang, which is a combination of two or more herbal prescriptions normally used to deal with more complicated disease patterns.

The Eight Precious Herbs Combination is a combination of the Four Major Herbs Combination and the Four Herbs Combination. It is used to deal with deficiency of both the Qi and blood, the signs and symptoms of which are a pale, or slightly yellowish complexion, palpitations, loss of appetite, shortness of breath, a reluctance to talk, fatigue in the extremities, dizziness, a pale tongue body and a thin weak pulse.

Herbal decotions TANG JI 汤剂

Boiling prescribed herbs or making a decoction is the most common and oldest method of preparing herbs. The history of herb decoction in China dates back to the time of the Xia Dynasty (2100 BC) approximately four thousand years ago, when copper vessels were widely used for culinary purposes and fermentation of spirits had been developed.

The invention of herbal decoction is attributed to a minister Yiyi 伊尹, who was in charge of decoctions and food preparations for the royal household during the Xia Dynasty. The boiling of herbs and the development of culinary skills were very closely intertwined at this early stage in China's history.

Before the advent of boiling herbs, individual herbs were masticated and then swallowed but once developed, it became possible to blend herbs and so blend their therapeutic actions. It also meant less toxicity in the oral administration of the herbs.

Boiling herbs is still the most popular method of preparing Chinese herbs for three reasons: 1. It is economical. 2. It is therapeutically flexible. 3. It is very efficient in extracting the herbs' therapeutic constituents.

The correct method of boiling herbs

There are three factors to consider when making herbal decoctions: the container, the water and the fire.

The ideal container used in boiling Chinese herbs is the clay pot because it has very stable chemical constituents, i.e. the material does not corrode in the boiling process, thereby ensuring the integrity of the decocted substances. Secondly, the heat conductibility of clay is very moderate so it spreads the heat very evenly.

Reinforced glass saucepans and porcelain-coated saucepans can also be used. Iron and copper saucepans should be not be used for decocting herbs for they corrode in the course of the boiling process and some herbs react with the metal.

Ordinary clear and clean tap drinking water can be used for decocting herbs but water containing high levels of heavy metals, pesticides, radiation waste or other impurities should never be used. The *Compendium of Materia Medica*, written during the time of the Ming Dynasty (1368–1644), prescribes 42 different types of water recommended for herb decoction, including spring, well, rain, river, snow, and dew water.

The amount of water used in a herb decoction is normally determined by the water-absorbing capacity of the herbs, the duration of boiling and the degree of heat used.

Generally speaking, in a packet of herbs one gram of herbs requires 10 millilitres of water. For example, in the prescription Honeysuckle Forsythia Combination the total weight of the herbs to be decocted amounts to 168 grams. Therefore the amount of water to be used is approximately 1680 millilitres of water. Normally, a packet of herbs is decocted twice, so 65 per cent of the water must be used in the first decoction, while the remaining 35 per cent is used in the second decoction.

The traditional way of measuring water was to lay all the dried herbs evenly in the container, add water to a height of 3–4 cm above the herbs, and if some of the herbs float in the water, then make a mark on the inner lining of the pot as to the height of the herb, then add more water.

Most Chinese herbs are dried substances of specific sizes and thicknesses. Before herbs are decocted, they are soaked in water to moisten and soften their tissues. Herbs with a very light texture and weight, like flowers, leaves and stems, need only about 20–30 minutes, while those with a heavy texture and weight, e.g. roots, rhizomes, seeds, fruits and minerals, have to be soaked for an hour. Soaking affords a maximum extraction of active therapeutic ingredients from the herbs' starches and proteins.

Through the process of osmosis the cells of the plants become turgid and inflated and these active ingredients within the cells dissolve and flow to the broader fluid tissue of the plant. When the soaked herbs are boiled, the heat bursts the tissues, releasing the proteins and starches into the decoction together with their active ingredients.

Boiling the herbs twice is one of the most efficient ways of maximising the extraction of their active ingredients. A study conducted in China, involving boiling the herbs in the Four Herbs Combination prescription confirmed that boiling herbs twice can result in a 70 to 80 per cent extraction of all the herbs' therapeutic ingredients.

In boiling herbs, the observation and regulation of heat or huo hou 火候 is a vital factor in ensuring a quality herb decoction. In many ways this is similar to the culinary art of cooking food.

For a herbal decoction, gas or electricity may be used. After soaking, put the herbs and water under a high heat. Once the water starts to boil, turn the heat to a 'gentle fire' or wen huo 文火, i.e. so it simmers. Stir the decoction once every seven minutes.

The duration of boiling depends upon the texture, weight and therapeutic nature of the herbs. Herbs consisting of roots, stems, fruits, marine shells, animal horns and scales, which are heavy and thick in texture and generally used for tonifying purposes, require a longer boiling duration for thorough extraction of the active ingredients. Usually the first boiling would require an hour of 'gentle fire' boiling; the second boiling, about half an hour of 'gentle fire' boiling. Herbs that are light in texture and weight and used for diaphoretic purposes, such as some flowers, leaves, and whole stalks, generally require only 10–15 minutes of 'gentle fire' boiling for the first boiling, followed by a second 5–10 minutes of 'gentle fire' boiling. As most of these herbs are rich in volatile oils, a shorter rather than longer boiling time is used to extract and prevent the loss of their aromatic, pungent and dispersing qualities.

As for those prescriptions which have a combination of light and heavy textured herbs, the first boiling would require 30 minutes of 'gentle fire' boiling, and 20 minutes of 'gentle fire' boiling for the second one.

After boiling the decoction, use a two-layered fine cotton cloth strainer to separate the residue from the decoction. Straining should be done immediately after boiling, while the decoction is still hot. This will ensure that certain compounds extracted during the boiling process are retained in the decoction and not form into large granules of sedimentation when the decoction turns cold. When straining the decoction, squeeze as much liquid out of the residue as possible. Straining the decoction also gets rid of some tiny substances like plant hair, which can be irritating when taken orally.

Oral administration of herbal decoction

The most common method of taking herb decoction is to mix together the two separate decoctions obtained by boiling the herbs twice and then divide this into two parts of 200–250 millilitres each, to be administered orally in one day. For the aged, physically weak or those with a prolonged illness, the decoction may be administered in a small dosage of, say, 150 millilitres each time.

Alternatively, the entire decoction from two boilings is mixed together and administered in full at one time. This type of administration is used for patients suffering from an acute or serious condition requiring rapid treatment. With this method the efficacy of the formula is stronger. In some instances, the herb decoction may be administered in full two or three times a day over a 24-hour period. A third option, recommended for patients who suffer from mouth or throat conditions, is to take the decoction several times a day or night in small quantities.

Generally speaking, the best time to administer a herbal decoction is in between meals, so as to avoid the mixing of food and decoction, which may affect the latter's efficacy. However, there are variations upon this rule. Taking the decoction on an empty stomach or ping dan fu 平旦服 is advised for patients who suffer from constipation or worms. Herb prescriptions which have a tonifying effect, like the Four Major Herbs Combination, must be taken before meals to enhance the full absorption of the medication. Herbal preparations which contain herbs irritating to the stomach may be taken after meals and those which calm the spirit and aid sleep, like the Sour Date Seed Combination, must be taken before going to bed. Lastly, herbal preparations which deal with exterior patterns (such as the common cold) may be taken any time.

Administering herb decoctions to children

Administering a herb decoction to children poses a big challenge to practitioners and parents alike with the taste and quantity of the decoction being a prominent consideration. The following points should be noted.

1. Concentrate the decoction. When boiling the decoction leave it for a longer period of time than usual under a gentle flame to allow more evaporation and so reduce the volume of the decoction. Generally speaking the dosage for children may be as follows:

a. For children of school age: 200–250 ml/day
b. For pre-school children: 150–200 ml/day
c. For infants: 60–100 ml/day
The above dose may be administered in small quantities several times.

2. For children who take the decoction of their own volition, a reward may be given such as fruit juices or fruit after taking the medication.

3. To infants or pre-school children administer only a few mouthfuls at a time followed by fruit sweets or fruit juices. Make sure you administer the medication slowly. For infants, hold their hands and head and keep them still. Then use a teaspoon to place the medication on the base of their tongue so that it can be swallowed naturally. Alternately, dip a sterile cotton wool ball into the decoction and then drip the decoction into the baby's mouth.

4. When administering herbal tablets or powders, you may mix these with soya milk and then feed the mixture to the child. Avoid mixing the decoction with animal milk as the protein in it may interact with active ingredients and so influence the therapeutic effect of the decoction.

Herbal decoction and food
Foods, like herbs, have certain natural inclinations and attributes, so the choice of food eaten should enhance the therapeutic qualities of the medication. In general terms, when taking herbal medication, avoid foods which are difficult to digest, specifically those which are irritating to the stomach, e.g. raw, cold, greasy, very rich or foul-smelling foods.

Patients with an internal heat pattern should avoid eating pungent-flavoured or peppery foods. Those with a damp and phlegm pattern should avoid rich, greasy and fatty foods. Those with itchy or other skin conditions, such as boils or sores, should avoid fish and prawns. Those with a deficient pattern and with a cold pathogen build-up should avoid cold foods and fruits. For certain allergy conditions, such as asthma or eczema, a person taking herbs should avoid eating chicken, fish, prawns, crabs, calamari, shellfish or any food which contains those proteins to which they are allergic. It is also not advisable to drink tea when taking medicinal decoctions.

Chinese herbal tablets and powders
Apart from decocted herbs, Chinese herbs also come in tablet and powder forms. These are especially suitable for people who find boiling herbs inconvenient. Tablets and powders come in set formulae referred to as 'formed medication' or 'cheng yao' 成药. Most of the herbal formulae discussed in this book have been manufactured into tablets or granulated powder. They may also be prepared simply as individual herbs, in which case specific herbs can be combined and tailored, like decoctions, to the clinical pattern of a particular patient.

There are two ways of manufacturing these tablets and powders. One method is to grind the dried herbs. This is a common method of manufacture in China. Another method is to decoct the herbs in large quantities. The decoctions are then freeze dried, like instant coffee. This form of manufacture is common in Japan and Taiwan.

CHINESE HERBAL PREPARATIONS WITH PHARMACEUTICAL INGREDIENTS (CHPPI)

Chinese herbal preparations with pharmaceutical ingredients (CHPPI) are 'formed medications' made from a combination of natural substances (plant, animal and/or minerals) and synthetic pharmaceutical substances. They come in standard pharmaceutical forms, such as sugar-coated tablets, injections, syrups and tinctures, or in traditional formed medications, such as pills and powders. People should be wary of consuming these substances.

A typical example of a CHPPI is a tablet for influenza and the common cold called 'Quick Relief Cold Tablets' or Gan Mao Su An Pian 感冒速安片. The main ingredients of this preparation are:

Rhubarb rhizome (*Rheum palmaturm*) or da huang 大黄
Cattle gall stone (*Calculus bovis*) or niu huang 牛黄
The steroid drug dexamethasone or di sai mi song 地塞米松

According to the Chinese technical literature (Zhu, 1991), this preparation works in accordance with the ingredients' pharmacological attributes. Rhubarb rhizome contains chemicals that can deactivate the influenza virus, while cattle gall stone has a sedating, antipyretic, anti-inflammatory and detoxifying effect. Combined, these two ingredients can be effective against upper respiratory tract infections, throat infections and mouth sores. Dexamethasone is a scheduled drug in Australia which can only be prescribed by Western medical practitioners, dentists or chemists. This corticosteroid has many effects, including toxic ones. Preparations such as these are best avoided.

CHPPI are mainly manufactured in China. They are an offspring of the interaction between TCM and Western medical knowledge which occurred in the late nineteenth and early twentieth century when scholars were advocating the pooling together of TCM and Western medicine. In China, CHPPI can be legally prescribed by TCM practitioners whose training includes the use of these preparations. CHPPI are now finding their way, albeit illegally, into Western countries like Australia, the USA and England. There have been reports of adverse reactions from the administration of these preparations. The use of these preparations in these countries is still an unsettled issue which needs to be dealt with in the future.

TOXICITY IN CHINESE HERBAL MEDICINE Du Xing 毒性

The question of toxicity, side effects and reactions to taking Chinese herbal medication is a question taken seriously by TCM practitioners and consumers alike. Statistics from China, while contradictory, confirm that this question is also a serious one in that country.

According to Guo, in *Dictionary of Toxic Herbs* (1992), within a two-year period, from 1988–1989, there were 400 cases of reported toxic reaction from taking herbs in China; out of these, 40 died. According to another source (Zhu, 1991) incomplete statistics confirm that in the 40 years from 1949 to 1989 at least 10,000 cases of toxic reactions to herbs, involving over 100 different types of herbs, occurred in China.

Outside China, there have also been cases of adverse reaction. In Australia, a recent case of severe reaction from the suspected administration of a herbal preparation containing the toxic herb aconite was reported.

The concept of toxicity or du xing in the course of TCM development has taken on a three-tiered meaning. First the name 'du' was used interchangeably with 'yao' the word for medicine or remedy in ancient times. Secondly, toxicity may be considered in terms of 'inclinations' of the Qi attribute and flavour of the medicinal substances. Thirdly, the term is understood in the English sense of poisonous and of producing adverse reactions. These reactions can be generalised into certain allergic reactions, such as skin itchiness and rash, to more severe reactions which affect normal physiological functions, e.g. digestive, respiratory, neurological, which can sometimes cause death.

Adverse reactions are not only restricted to toxic herbs but can also include non-toxic ones which have been improperly used due to a wrongly prescribed dosage or herb.

Tan (1990) identified 348 cases of adverse reactions to medicinal herbs in China over 30 years resulting in nine deaths (Tan, 1990). Of these fatalities, four were due to overdoses, while two were due to a wrongly prescribed herbs. The herbs which caused these nine fatalities were:

1. *Phytolacca acinosa* (Shang lu 商陆)
2. *Cucumis melo* (stem) (Ku ding Xiang 苦丁香)
3. *Hyoscyamus niger* (tian xian zi 天仙子)
4. *Strychnos wallichiana* (ma qian zi 马前子)
5. *Typhonium giganteum* (du jiao lian 独角莲)
6. Dried skin secretion of toad (chan su 蟾酥)
7. *Strychnos ignatii* (lu song guo 吕宋果)

In 1983, 200 people developed adverse reactions from taking an anti-flu herbal preparation which contained the toxic herb *Sophora subprostrata* (guang dou gen 广豆根). This herb was erroneously mistaken for another herb. The reactions included headache, abdominal pain, nausea, vomiting, body chills, shaking, tremors, hypertension and rapid heart rate.

This survey also reported 26 cases of allergic reactions to the taking of non-toxic Chinese herbs. These ranged from skin rashes and itchiness, to respiratory problems, e.g. wheezing and hurried breathing, to abdominal problems, eg. diarrhoea, and to more severe urological and neurological reactions. The survey did not indicate whether the patients involved had a history of allergy.

The non-toxic herbs implicated in these allergic reactions included tangerine peel, *Ramus loranthi parasiticus* (sang ji sheng), sour date seeds, China root (fu ling), loquat leaf (pi ba ye), *Trichosanthes kirlowii* (tian hua fen), *Brucea javanica* (ya dan zi), *Magnolia liliflora* (xin yi), Dandelion (pu gong ying), Ginseng, *Arctium lappa* (niu bang zi), *Commiphora myrrha* (mo yao), *Inula britannica* (xuan fu hua), *Acorus gramineus* (shi chang pu).

In 1979, the Chinese government imposed restrictions on the use of a number of toxic herbs and substances. As a result the following toxic herbs cannot be obtained over the counter without a TCM doctor's prescription and with an official seal on it :

1. Raw *Aconite carmichaeli* (sheng fu zi 生附子)

2. Raw *Strychnos wallichiana* (sheng ma qian zi 生马前子)

3. Raw *Radix aconiti* (sheng wu tou 生乌头)

4. Raw *Aconitum kusnezofii* (sheng cao wu 生草乌)

5. *Mylabris phalerata* (ban mao 斑蝥)

6. *Epicauta hirticornis* (ge shang ting zhang 葛上亭长)

7. *Meloe crvinus Marseul* (di dan 地胆)

8. Raw *Croton tiglium* (sheng ba dou 生巴豆)

9. Raw *Pinella ternata* (sheng ban xia 生半夏)

10. Raw *Rhizoma arisaematis* (sheng nan xing 生南星)

11. Raw *Euphorbia kansui* (sheng gan sui 生甘遂)

12. *Datura stramonium* (yang jin hua 洋金花)

13. Raw *Euphorbia lathyris* (sheng qian jin zi 生千金子)

14. Raw *Hyoscyamus niger* (sheng tian xian zi 生天仙子)

15. Toad skin secretion (chan su 蟾酥)

Many of these would be classified in Western medicine as very poisonous. Some, such as aconite, can lead to death.

There is no unified school of thought in China about what constitutes 'toxic' herbs or substances. However, some TCM academics and researchers are starting to define the degrees of toxic reactions from medicinal substances. In their research so far, 503 toxic herbs and substances have been identified; of these, 420 are plants, 50 are animal byproducts and 33 are minerals. These toxic herbs and substances have been ranked into four categories of toxicity.

HERB PROCESSING *Pao Zhi* 炮制

Before Chinese herbs can be used for decoction or manufactured into tablets or powders, they must be processed. This processing is called pao zhi 炮制 Processing may include cleaning, washing or drying. It may also entail an elaborate process of soaking in water, frying in vinegar, honey or salt, or toasting. Once a particular herb has undergone processing it is graded in accordance with its quality and packaged into small quantities. This finished product is referred to as 'yin pian' 饮片 or 'herb slices ready for ingestion'.

The processing of herbs can have the effect of enhancing or changing the therapeutic inclinations of herbs, as well as tempering their toxicity. The use of spirits and wine in processing dangui root, for example, is done to enhance its dispersing qualities, and ginger is used in the processing of the herb *Pinella ternata* or ban xia in order to enhance its anti-emetic qualities. Similarly toasting the root of *Rehmannia glutinosa* or sheng di huang in wine or spirits can change its cooling Qi attributes into a warm attribute.

In the case of herbs with toxic side effects, subjecting them to heat, soaking them in water or mixing them with other substances can temper or reduce the side effects. This is another reason why *Pinella ternata* is mixed with ginger in the above mentioned example.

In China the processing of the toxic herb *Aconite carmichaeli* involves soaking it in water for a long period of time to hydrolyse the toxic compound, aconitine, into a non-toxic compound, aconine, thereby lessening the toxicity of the herb itself (Qi, 1987).

FOOD THERAPY
食疗

FOOD THERAPY OR SHI LIAO IS A BODY OF TCM KNOWLEDGE WHICH USES varieties of grains, fruits, vegetables, meat, seafoods, condiments, nuts and herbs, and their combinations, to maintain health and to prevent and treat illness. Like herbs, each food's therapeutic inclinations has been defined in the course of its protracted use in addressing clinical patterns. In TCM, food has been enlisted as an ally in the fight against disease and illness.

Food is one of man's inseparable links with nature. For several thousands of years, Chinese medical scholars have seen food as a harmonising agent, endowed with certain natural attributes vital for redressing disharmony both within and between oneself and the natural forces. TCM holds that since food and medicinal herbs have similar origins, food can be used as medicine and vice-versa. A clear example of this is ginger which is both a common medicinal ingredient and common culinary recipe ingredient.

Normal food does not produce unfavourable side effects, whereas potent medicinal herbs must be taken with caution. Since therapeutic food is very safe, it can be considered as the best form of medicine. Ancient medical scholars held that food should be used to regulate body functions and tonify what is weak and deficient, while individual remedies, such as medicinal herbs, acupuncture and tuina, must be used to meet the illness head on. A Tang-dynasty medical scholar, Sun Zi Miao, devoted a whole chapter to food therapy in his medical classic, *Prescriptions Worth A Thousand Gold Ducats*. He said, 'Use food to cure it (illness). If food does not work, then use other medicinal remedies.'

FOOD INCLINATIONS — THE THERAPEUTIC ATTRIBUTES OF FOODS

As in the case of medicinal herbs and substances, foods possess various inclinations, such as Qi attributes, flavours, channel associations and therapeutic actions. Over 2000 years, hundreds of varieties of foods have been categorised in accordance with these criteria.

Food Qi Attributes

The Qi attribute of food can be cold, cool, hot, warm or neutral. Such attributes refer to body temperature responses when we eat certain foods and to the effects of these in harmonising extremes of cold or hot clinical patterns.

Foods which have a hot or warm Qi attribute produce a hot or warm body sensation when eaten, digested and absorbed by the body. They accordingly redress cold clinical patterns. Examples of these foods are ginger, garlic, cherries, mutton and walnuts. Conversely, foods with a cold and cool Qi, induce a cold and cooling sensation when eaten and redress hot clinical patterns. Examples are bananas, papaws, watermelons, cucumbers, tea, mung beans and bean curd. Foods with a neutral Qi, which are neither hot, warm, cool nor cold, have a moderating effect upon the body.

Food Flavours

A particular food can have one of five flavours: sour, bitter, sweet, pungent or salty. In some cases, a particular food may have two flavours. For example, an apple has both a sour and a sweet flavour. Food flavours or wei 味 in the context of TCM, are defined both by taste, as differentiated by the taste buds, and by a flavour's harmonising effects on clinical patterns.

Food with a sour or puckery flavour has a gathering or astringent effect which can stop profuse sweating, diarrhoea and other uncontrollable body fluid secretions. Smoked plum (prune) juice, for example, taken during the hot summer season prevents excessive sweating.

Pungent-tasting foods produce the opposite effect to sour foods. They promote the flow of Qi and blood within the channels and have a dispersing and moistening effect, opening the skin pores and inducing perspiration. Examples are ginger, spring onions, garlic and pepper. Wine and other forms of spirits also possess pungent flavours. For common colds manifesting an exterior wind-cold clinical pattern, the main symptoms of which are body chills and bone and joint pains, a hot rice porridge mixed with several slices of ginger is recommended (a common recipe in the average Chinese household). The pungent tasting ginger is used to disperse the cold pathogenic factor affecting the surface of the body, the cause of this clinical pattern.

Sweet-flavoured foods have a tonifying and nourishing effect and relieve spasms. Hence they are used to deal with deficient clinical patterns. A typical example of a sweet-flavoured food with a tonifying effect is the chestnut. Its warm Qi attribute deals with the clinical pattern of kidney Qi deficiency, the signs and symptoms which are lower back pains, weakness of the knees and frequent urination. Other examples of food with sweet flavour are grapes, papaws, rice, bean curd (tofu), mutton and prawns.

A combination of a sour and sweet flavour leads to the combined effect of nourishing the body essence or jing, and moistening dryness. This is termed 'sweet and sour flavour beneficial to the yin constitutional essence'. Rice vinegar boiled with tofu to treat diarrhoea is a typical example. Rice vinegar has a sour flavour and thus an astringent effect, while tofu with a sweet flavour can tonify the Qi.

Bitter-tasting food produces a downward draining effect, deals with hot clinical patterns and dries dampness and mucus in the body. For example, tea of any variety, which is a bitter-tasting food, can clear heat from the eyes and head, quench thirst, alleviate irritability, aid digestion and act as a diuretic.

Salty-flavoured foods can soften and dissolve the accumulation of a hard mass resulting from heat and phlegm, e.g. goitre and inflamed lymphatic nodes. Most marine products fall into this category. A good example is the sea cucumber, which is salty in flavour with a warm Qi attribute. It is an excellent food for tonifying kidney system deficiencies, nourishing the blood and moistening dryness. When cooked with mutton (hot Qi attribute and sweet flavour), it can be a good supplementary diet for people suffering from low sexual libido and impotency. Another example of salty food is clam, which with its diuretic effect is helpful for treating fluid retention.

COMMON FOODS, THEIR INCLINATIONS AND APPLICATIONS

Vegetables

Celery *Oenanthe javanica* Qin Cai 芹菜

Qi Attribute:	Cool
Flavour:	Sweet and pungent
Therapeutic Action:	Drains heat and promotes urination
Food Therapy Application:	1. Hypertension: 1/2 cup of juice of the young celery stem. Drink twice a day.
	2. Diabetes: 500 g of boiled celery juice every day.
	3. Pain and incontinence during urination: drink juice of the white root of the celery stem.

Note: It is best to eat the tender stems of the celery. Regular eating of celery can drain heat among patients with a yin deficiency and a hyperactive fire clinical pattern. However, it is not advisable for those with spleen and stomach deficiency clinical patterns and diarrhoea to eat too much.

Tomato *Lycopersicon esculentum* Xi hong shi 西红柿

Qi Attribute:	Slightly cold
Flavour:	Sweet and sour
Therapeutic Action:	Promotes body fluid production and stops thirst, tonifies the stomach system and aids digestion
Food Therapy Application:	1. Thirst when convalescing from severe fever conditions: tomato juice (without seed and peeled) with white sugar.

2. Loss of appetite due to summer heat: eat some tomatoes which have been stir-fried in vegetable oil with added broth.

Bok Choy (Chinese Cabbage) *Brassica chinensis* Bai Cai 白菜

Qi Attribute:	Slightly cold
Flavour:	Sweet
Therapeutic Action:	Drains heat and promotes urination, nurtures the stomach organ system and detoxifies
Food Therapy Application:	1. Bok choy can be used as a supplementary diet for a patient with a clinical pattern of stomach yin deficiency generating heat, the signs and symptoms of which are a dry mouth with loss of appetite or a cough with phlegm expectoration, blocked urination etc.
	2. Eaten raw, it can be used as an alcohol detoxification agent.
	3. Constipation: Stir-fry 1/4 kg bok choy and eat everyday.

Carrots *Oaucus carota* Hu Luo Bo 胡萝卜

Qi Attribute:	Neutral
Flavour:	Sweet
Therapeutic Action:	Tonifies a spleen system deficiency, facilitates Qi circulation and aids digestion
Food Therapy Application:	1. For old and young patients with physical debility: When eaten cooked, carrots can tonify the Qi and promote blood production.
	2. Can address spleen Qi deficiency clinical patterns with food stagnation, the signs and symptoms of which are chest and abdominal congestion, loss of appetite and chronic diarrhoea.

Lettuce *Lactuca sativa* Wo Ju 莴苣

Qi Attribute:	Slightly cold
Flavour:	Bitter and sweet
Therapeutic Action:	Drains heat and loosens phlegm, facilitates Qi circulation and decongests the chest
Food Therapy Application:	1. When eaten raw or cooked, lettuce can drain

phlegm from the chest. It can be eaten as a supplementary food in the clinical pattern of heat in the chest and diaphragm, with signs and symptoms of cough with a lot of phlegm expectoration, difficulty in urination and defecation, and blood in the urine.

2. Lettuce can also facilitate the circulation of Qi and blood thereby removing blockage in the channels. It may be eaten as a supplementary food for food stagnation, as well as for stagnation in the flow of Qi and blood, with symptoms of chest congestion and loss of appetite. In this sense, lettuce can also treat stagnated lactation.

Grain

White Polished Rice *Oryza sativa* Jing Mi 粳米

Qi Attribute:	Neutral
Flavour:	Sweet
Therapeutic Action:	Tonifies the spleen system, moderates the stomach system functions, benefits the body's constitutional essence or jing and strengthens the will
Food Therapy Application:	1. Rice lightens the body, promotes good facial colour and improves hearing and vision.
	2. Rice can regulate the stomach Qi and stop diarrhoea. It can tonify a spleen system deficiency characterised by chest and abdominal congestion, loss of appetite, diarrhoea and thinning of the muscular tissues.

Oatmeal *Avena sativa* Yan Mai 燕麦

Qi Attribute:	Neutral
Flavour:	Sweet
Therapeutic Action:	Tonifies deficient spleen and stomach systems. Promotes intestinal movements and hastens childbirth
Food Therapy Application:	1. When boiled to make porridge, it can promote intestinal movement and so alleviate constipation. Oatmeal porridge can also hasten childbirth.

2. Oatmeal porridge can tonify deficient spleen and stomach systems, thereby enhancing appetite and body energy.

Mung Bean *Rhasealus radiatus* Lu Dou 绿豆

Qi Attribute:	Cold
Flavour:	Sweet
Therapeutic Action:	Drains heat and detoxifies, promotes body fluid production, urination and eliminates body fluid retention

Food Therapy Application:
1. Boiled mung beans, taken as soup with a little sugar, can promote urination and so treat fluid retention
2. Boiled mung beans dispel extreme heat and cool the body, especially during summer. They can be used as a supplementary diet in dealing with skin conditions in the category of wind-heat clinical patterns.
3. Ground mung beans or boiled mung bean soup has been used in China to deal with carbon monoxide poisoning resulting from coal emissions, and alcohol poisoning. Also useful for poisoning from plants, especially when combined with licorice.

Soya Beans *Glycine max* Huang Dou 黄豆

Qi Attribute:	Neutral
Flavour:	Sweet
Therapeutic Action:	Tonifies the spleen system, cools heat and detoxifies

Food Therapy Application:
1. Boiled soya bean or soya milk can tonify the spleen system and strengthen the body. It is an ideal tonifying food, recommended for conditions of physical debility, lack of energy and problems with lactation due to physical debility.
2. Soya milk can also be good for infants who suffer from diarrhoea due to inability to absorb food nutrients.

Wheat *Triticum aestivum* Xiao Mai 小麦

Qi Attribute:	Neutral
Flavour:	Sweet
Therapeutic Action:	Tonifies the heart system, dispels heat and quenches thirst

Food Therapy Application:
1. Wheat flour made into baked or steamed bread can tonify the heart system and thus alleviate restlessness and sleeplessness.
2. Dryness in the mouth and thirst: drink teas boiled with 30–69 g wheat grain.
3. Tonifies the five organ systems and thickens the stomach and intestines. Wheat, eaten as boiled grain or made into steamed or baked bread, can alleviate diarrhoea, with shortness of breath and physical debility.

Fruits

Banana *Musa paradisiaca* Xiang Jiao 香蕉

Qi Attribute:	Cold
Flavour:	Sweet
Therapeutic Action:	Drains heat and promotes body fluid production, moistens the intestines

Food Therapy Application:
1. Ripe bananas can drain heat from the lungs and spleen systems, promote body fluid production, quench thirst, moisten the lungs and enhance intestinal movements. They can be recommended as a supplementary fruit for patients with a very high fever and constipation. Bananas can also be beneficial for haemorrhoids. Unripe bananas are slightly astringent, and can reduce diarrhoea.

Grapes *Vitis vinifera* Pu Tao 葡萄

Qi Attribute:	Neutral
Flavour:	Sweet and sour
Therapeutic Action:	Tonifies deficient Qi and blood, strengthens the tendons and bones, promotes urination

Food Therapy Application:
1. Grapes tonify the kidney and liver systems and specifically address liver and kidney yin defi-

ciency clinical patterns, characterised by palpitations and night sweats, a dry cough, lower back pains and tendon and bone weakness.

2. Grapes tonify Qi and blood deficiency and promote urination. They address a spleen deficiency clinical pattern with symptoms of shortness of breath, physical weakness, coughing with white phlegm, fluid retention in the face and extremities and urinary difficulties.

Lemon *Citrus limon* Ning Meng 柠檬

Qi Attribute:	Neutral
Flavour:	Sour
Therapeutic Action:	Promotes the production of body fluids and settles foetus
Food Therapy Application:	1. Lemon juice taken during summer can alleviate internal body heat.
	2. Lemon juice can settle the foetus in cases of threatened abortion.

Nashi Pear *Pyrus bretschneideri* Bai Li 白梨

Qi Attribute:	Cold
Flavour:	Sweet and slightly sour
Therapeutic Action:	Nourishes the yin and drains heat, moistens the lung system and stops coughing
Food Therapy Application:	1. Nashi pear can alleviate coughing as one of the symptoms of a lung dryness clinical pattern with other symptoms of a dry throat, red eyes, hurried breathing and wheezing.
	2. Fresh nashi pear can be used to nourish the body in the later stages of fever related conditions.

Apple *Malus pumila* Ping Guo 苹果

Qi Attribute:	Cool
Flavour:	Sweet
Therapeutic Action:	Tonifies deficient spleen and stomach, promotes body fluid production and moistens body dryness
Food Therapy Application:	1. Eat fresh apples when there are clinical patterns of spleen and stomach deficiency, e.g. lack of spirit, loss of appetite and sluggish digestion.

2. Fresh apple juice can promote body fluid production, opens the stomach and moistens the lungs to address the clinical pattern characterised by irritability, thirst, cough and night sweats.

Meat

Mutton *Ovis aries* Yang Rou 羊肉

Qi Attribute:	Warm
Flavour:	Sweet
Therapeutic Action:	Tonifies deficient Qi and nourishes the blood, warms the middle and lower energiser (see glossary)
Food Therapy Application:	1. Cooked mutton can tonify the Qi and nourish the blood. Patients suffering from heavy menstrual bleeding, physical debility as a result of prolonged illness and consumptive illness should eat more mutton. Mutton should be avoided when there are signs of a hot clinical pattern.
	2. Mutton broth can be beneficial for patients with vomiting and diarrhoea resulting from a deficient and cold clinical pattern, and for women with post-partum pain accompanied by a feeling of coldness in the abdominal area.

Venison *Cervus nippon* Lu Rou 鹿肉

Qi Attribute:	Warm
Flavour:	Sweet
Therapeutic Action:	Tonifies deficient spleen Qi, warms the yang of the kidney system
Food Therapy Application:	1. The meat or the broth can address clinical patterns of deficiency of kidney yang system with symptoms of weakness in the low back and knees, impotency or seminal emission, coldness in the testicles, dizziness and ringing in the ear.
	2. Venison is a good tonic for the spleen system. Eaten as a dish, it can address the clinical pattern of a deficient spleen Qi system, e.g. loss

of weight, shortness of breath, feeling of fatigue, loss of appetite.

3. Venison benefits all the five organ systems and the bones and tendons of a healthy person.

Beef *Bos taurus domesticus* Niu Rou 牛肉

Qi Attribute:	Neutral
Flavour:	Sweet
Therapeutic Action:	Tonifies deficient spleen Qi, softens phlegm and dispels wind
Food Therapy Application:	1. Beef is another food tonic. Eating it as a dish can address a spleen Qi deficiency clinical pattern, the symptoms of which are loss of weight after prolonged illness, poor appetite, soreness and weakness in the back and knees and fluid retention.
	2. When eaten by healthy people, beef tonifies the Qi and strengthens the body physically.

Pork *Sus scrofa domestica* Zhu Rou 猪肉

Qi Attribute:	Neutral
Flavour:	Sweet and salty
Therapeutic Action:	Nourishes the yin constitutional essence and moistens dryness
Food Therapy Application:	1. Eaten as a dish, pork can tonify the kidney system to benefit the constitutional essence and nourish the liver system to benefit the blood. Hence it can tonify a deficient clinical pattern of the kidney system characterised by prolonged illness and blood deficiency after childbirth.
	2. Cold, fat-free pork broth can address body fluid loss resulting from a prolonged feverish condition.

Chicken Meat *Gallus gallus domesticus* Ji Rou 鸡肉

Qi Attribute:	Warm
Flavour:	Sweet
Therapeutic Action:	Warms the middle energiser, tonifies the Qi, tonifies the constitutional essence jing and fills the bone marrow

Food Therapy Application: 1. A healthy person who eats chicken can replenish their strength and strengthen their body.

2. Chicken and its broth are excellent tonic foods. They address deficient clinical patterns which are characterised by loss of weight, loss of appetite, diarrhoea, fluid retention, frequent urination, excessive vaginal discharge, excessive menstrual bleeding and limited lactation after birth.

Marine Products

Prawn *Penaeus orientalis* Dui Xia 对虾

Qi Attribute: Warm
Flavour: Sweet and salty
Therapeutic Action: Tonifies deficient yang of the kidney system, tonifies the Qi and opens the stomach
Food Therapy Application: 1. Prawns, stir-fried with wine and then eaten as a dish, can deal with impotency brought on by a kidney yang deficiency clinical pattern.

2. A healthy person who eats cooked prawns can strengthen their body and increase their energy.

3. Cooked prawns can also tonify deficient kidney and spleen systems with a clinical pattern characterised by physical debility resulting from prolonged illness, shortness of breath and physical weakness, loss of appetite, loss of weight and pale complexion.

Oysters *Ostrea gigas* Mu Li 牡蛎

Qi Attribute: Neutral
Flavour: Sweet and salty
Therapeutic Action: Nourishes the yin constitutional essence and blood, drains heat and detoxifies
Food Therapy Application: This is a food tonic which can nourish a deficient blood and yin clinical pattern with symptoms of restlessness, inability to get to sleep, and thirst and feverish sensations after drinking alcohol.

Abalone *Haliotis diversicolor* Bao Yu 鲍鱼

Qi Attribute:	Neutral
Flavour:	Sweet and salty
Therapeutic Action:	Nourishes the yin and benefits the essence, drains heat and dampness

Food Therapy Application: 1. Abalone can nourish the yin constitutional essence, tonify deficiencies and benefit vision. Eating abalone can address a yin deficiency internal heat clinical pattern with symptoms of dry cough, failing vision, profuse menstrual bleeding etc.
2. Cooked abalone and broth can drain heat and dampness and address an internal heat and dampness clinical pattern with symptoms of urinary difficulties, thick and yellow vaginal discharge and skin conditions which will not heal.

Crab Meat *Eriocheir sinensis* Xie Rou 蟹肉

Qi Attribute:	Cold
Flavour:	Sweet
Therapeutic Action:	Tonifies the yin and the marrow, drains heat and softens phlegm, nourishes the tendons and facilitates blood flow.

Food Therapy Application: 1. Crab meat as a dish can address a liver and kidney system deficiency clinical pattern with symptoms of lower back pain, wobbly knees, dizziness and forgetfulness.
2. The cold Qi attribute of crab meat means it can deal with an internal heat and phlegm clinical pattern with symptoms of facial swelling and throat swelling and pain.

Condiments

Fresh Ginger *Zingiber officinale* Xian Jiang 鲜姜

Qi Attribute:	Warm
Flavour:	Pungent
Therapeutic Action:	Stops vomiting, softens phlegm, promotes sweating

Food Therapy Application: 1. For vomiting, mix one spoonful of ginger juice with some sugar and water. Boil and drink 4–5 times a day.
2. Common cold with a wind-cold pattern: mix 5 slices of ginger with some brown sugar and water. Boil and drink while still warm.

Food	Qi attributes					Flavour				
	Cold	Cool	Warm	Hot	Neutral	Sour	Bitter	Sweet	Pungent	Salty
Symbol	★	+	#	%	=	0	b	e	p	@
Fruit										
Apple					=	0		e		
Apricot			#			0		e		
Bananas	★							e		
Cherry			#			0		e		
Dates					=			e		
Grapes					=	0		e		
Longans					=			e		
Lychees			#			0		e		
Mango					=	0		e		
Papaw	★							e		
Peach			#			0		e		
Smoked plums					=	0				
Pomelo	★					0		e		
Tangerine		+				0		e		
Watermelon	★							e		
Vegetables										
Pear Bitter gourd	★					0				
Carrot					=			e		
Bamboo shoots	★							e	p	
Celery		+						e	p	
Chilli				%					p	
Chinese cabbage	★				=			e		

Food	Qui attributes					Flavour				
	Cold	Cool	Warm	Hot	Neutral	Sour	Bitter	Sweet	Pungent	Salty
Symbol	★	+	#	%	=	0	b	e	p	@

Vegetable (contd)

Food	Cold	Cool	Warm	Hot	Neutral	Sour	Bitter	Sweet	Pungent	Salty
Cucumber	★							e		
Edible fungus					=			e		
Eggplant		+						e		
Garlic			#						p	
Ginger			#						p	
Laver	★							e		@
Lettuce		+					b	e		
Mushroom		+						e		
Potato					=			e		
Pumpkin		+						e		
Rice					=			e		
Vinegar			%			0				
Seaweed	★									@
Spinach		+						e		
Spring onions			%						p	
Tomato	★					0		e		
Tea	★						b	e		

Grain, Nuts

Food	Cold	Cool	Warm	Hot	Neutral	Sour	Bitter	Sweet	Pungent	Salty
Chestnut			#					e		@
Glutinous rice				%				e		
Maize					=			e		
Mung bean	★							e		
Pine nut				%				e		
Red bean					=	0		e		
Rice					=			e		
Wheat		+						e		
Soya been					=			e		
Bean curd		+						e		
Walnut				%				e		

Food	Qui attributes					Flavour				
	Cold	Cool	Warm	Hot	Neutral	Sour	Bitter	Sweet	Pungent	Salty
Symbol	★	+	#	%	=	0	b	e	p	@
Grain, Nuts (contd)										
Peanut					=			e		
Pepper				%					p	
Sesame seeds					=			e		
Soya milk					=			e		
Meat & Marine Products										
Abalone				%						@
Beef				%	=			e		
Chicken				%	=			e		
Carp				%				e		
Clam					=					@
Crab	★									@
Cuttlefish					=					@
Duck		+						e		
Egg (chicken)					=			e		
Honey					=			e		
Cow's milk					=			e		
Mussels				%						@
Mutton			#					e		
Pork					=			e		@
Prawns				%				e		
Oyster	★									@
Quail					=			e		
Sea cucumber				%						@
Venison				%						@

• C H A P T E R   V I •

THE PRACTICE OF ACUPUNCTURE
针灸

IN CHINESE, ACUPUNCTURE IS WRITTEN IN TWO CHARACTERS: 'ZHEN' 针 AND 'jiu' 灸. Zhen refers to the acupuncture needle; jiu refers to moxibustion, a procedure in which a compressed herb, e.g. mugwort, is burned over an acupuncture point (acupoint) to produce heat. Acupuncture therefore involves inserting needles into acupoints and moxibustion.

To understand acupuncture, its practice has to be put into the context of the whole TCM practice, its philosophy and the many procedures which constitute this ancient technology.

ACUPUNCTURE POINTS *XUE WEI* 穴位

There are approximately 2000 acupoints or mapped areas on the body's surface, each with a name and an internationally recognised alphanumeric code. The points have a diameter of five to ten millimetres and an average depth of 17.9 mm. There are 365 commonly used acupoints which join like dots and dashes on the surface of the body to form a network of linear conduits termed acupuncture channels or meridians.

According to the ancient acupuncture channel theory, these networks or conduits connect the surface of the body with the various internal organ systems. Acupoints located along the meridians are termed 'channel points', while the rest are termed 'off-channel acupuncture points'.

Once the needle's tip is inserted into any of these acupoints, a stimulus is triggered and a peculiar sensation is felt, which is a composite sensory perception that is a blending or accentuation of a localised sensation of numbness, soreness, swelling, heaviness or slight pain. A radiating sensation which extends towards a definite direction and length can also sometimes be felt. This phenomenon is referred to as acupuncture sensation or 'de Qi' which means the arrival of the Qi. The therapeutic effect from acupuncture is contingent upon the patient feeling this Qi.

Every acupoint or combination thereof has a therapeutic action or gong xiao which can deal with specific clinical patterns. This is determined by each acupoint's channel and internal organ system association, its specific location on the surface of the body, and the type of stimulus applied to it.

THE ACUPUNCTURE CHANNEL NETWORK
JING LUO 经络

Acupoints constitute the dots and dashes on the surface of the body, whereas acupuncture meridians or channels are the linear structures which link these points into an intricate network connecting with the body's internal organ systems. In Chinese, acupuncture channels are referred to as 'jing luo'. 'Jing' means a pathway which runs up and down and connects the inner and outer, while 'luo' means a network which intersects and covers all areas of the body. Thus together, these words mean 'a network of pathways'.

Upon discovery of the therapeutic functions of acupuncture points vis-a-vis clinical patterns, ancient medical scholars also discovered sensory links between acupoints on the surface of the body and the normal and abnormal functioning of internal organ systems inside the body. On the basis of this observed sensory experience, ancient medical scholars used certain philosophical concepts, e.g. the philosophy of the yin and yang, to develop the workings and theory of the acupuncture channel system.

The first ancient medical text to document the acupuncture meridian network was the second volume of the *Yellow Emperor's Canons On Medicine*, the *Canon On Acupuncture*, written during the period of the Warring States (475–221 BC). According to this canon, the network of channels is a web of pathways that links the internal organ system with the skin, flesh, ligaments and bones, making the body function as an integral whole. Connecting the internal, external, lower and outer parts of the body, the network channels and transports Qi, blood and body fluids to all parts of the body, thereby providing them with nourishment. If the network of the channels functions normally, then the Qi, blood and body fluids can flow smoothly to the internal organ systems, bringing nourishment to them and making the body free from illness. However, if any part of the channel system becomes blocked or weak and deficient, disease occurs and clinical patterns corresponding to the blocked channel(s) will be manifested. Most clinical patterns correspond to the signs and symptoms occurring along the orbit flow of the blocked channels. For example, pain along the flanks or localised tenderness along this region reflects disharmony of the liver system whose channel flows through these regions.

There are seven interconnected networks of acupuncture meridians that have been explored and mapped out. These are:

1. The Twelve Regular Channels
2. The Eight Extra Channels
3. The Twelve Divergent Channels
4. The Fifteen Collaterals
5. The Minute Connecting Channels
6. The Twelve Tendon Channels
7. The Twelve Cutaneous Channels

For clinical purposes the most important among the above channel networks are the Twelve Regular Channels and two of the Eight Extra Channels. The 365 commonly used acupoints are all located along these channels as they criss-cross the surface of the body.

Each of the Twelve Regular Channels is named in accordance with the internal organ system with which it is connected, its yin and yang categorisation and whether it runs along the upper or lower extremities. There are in all six visceral organ systems (the heart, liver, spleen, lungs, kidneys and pericardium) and six hollow organ systems (the small intestine, gall bladder, stomach, large intestine, urinary bladder and triple energiser). Each of the Twelve Regular Channels connects with one visceral and one hollow organ system, making six channels paired to one another. These are:

Yin Channels	**Yang Channels**
Upper Extremities	
1. Hand Greater Yin Lung Channel	Hand Bright Yang Large Intestine Channel
2. Hand Lesser Yin Heart Channel	Hand Greater Yang Small Intestine Channel
3. Hand Terminal Yin Pericardium Channel	Hand Lesser Yang Triple Energiser Channel
Lower Extremities	
4. Foot Greater Yin Spleen Channel	Foot Bright Yang Stomach Channel
5. Foot Lesser Yin Kidney Channel	Foot Greater Yang Urinary Bladder Channel
6. Foot Terminal Yin Liver Channel	Foot Lesser Yang Gall Bladder Channel

The yin channels connect with the visceral organ systems and flow along the inner side of the extremities, while the yang channels connect with the hollow organ systems and flow along the lateral and outer areas of the extremities.

In accordance with the ebb and flow of yin Qi or yang Qi, the yin and yang channels are further subdivided into three types. The channel where the yin Qi is just beginning to flow is the Lesser Yin Channel, where there is a preponderance of yin Qi is the Greater Yin Channel; where the yin Qi has waned to its lowest point is the Terminal Yin Channel.

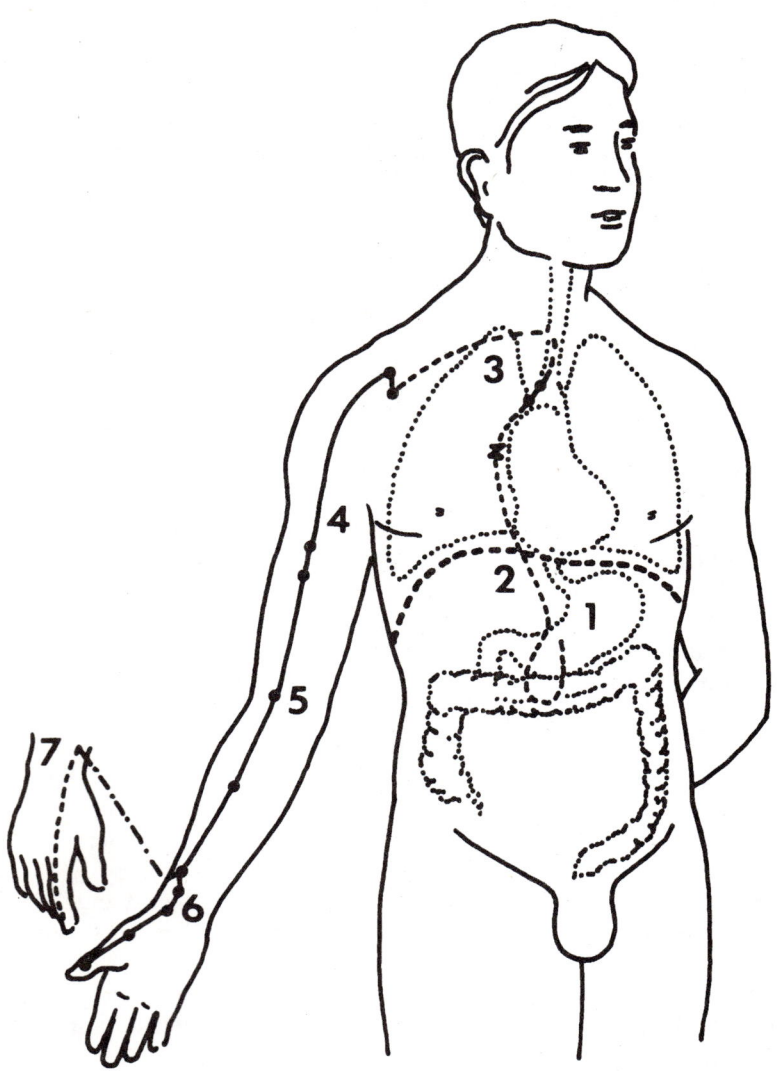

Hand Greater Yin Lung Channel

(Numbers indicate the direction of the flow of the Qi.)

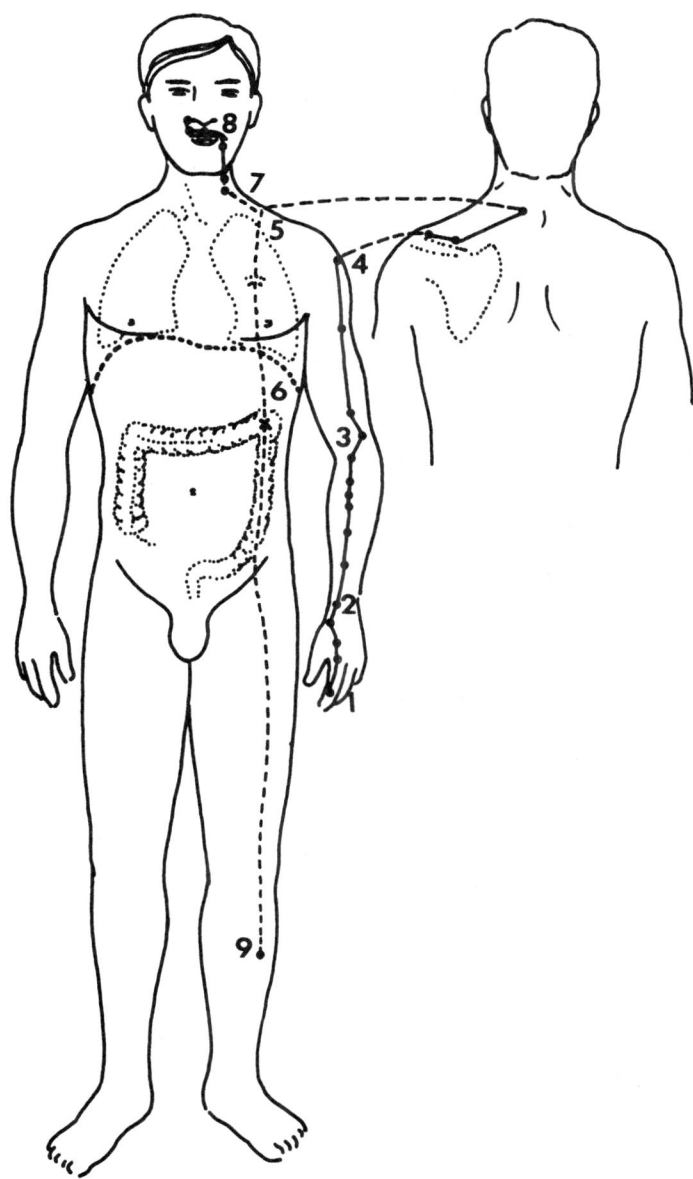

Hand Bright Yang Large Intestine Channel

(Numbers indicate the direction of the flow of the Qi.)

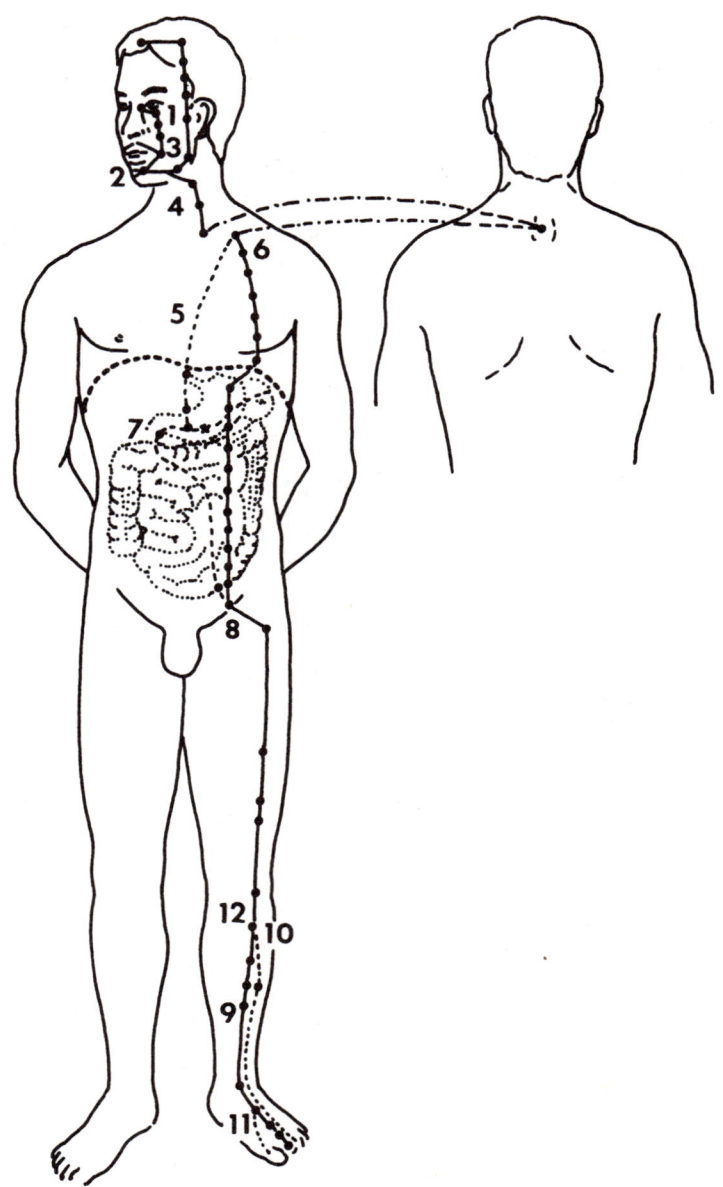

Foot Bright Yang Stomach Channel

(Numbers indicate the direction of the flow of the Qi.)

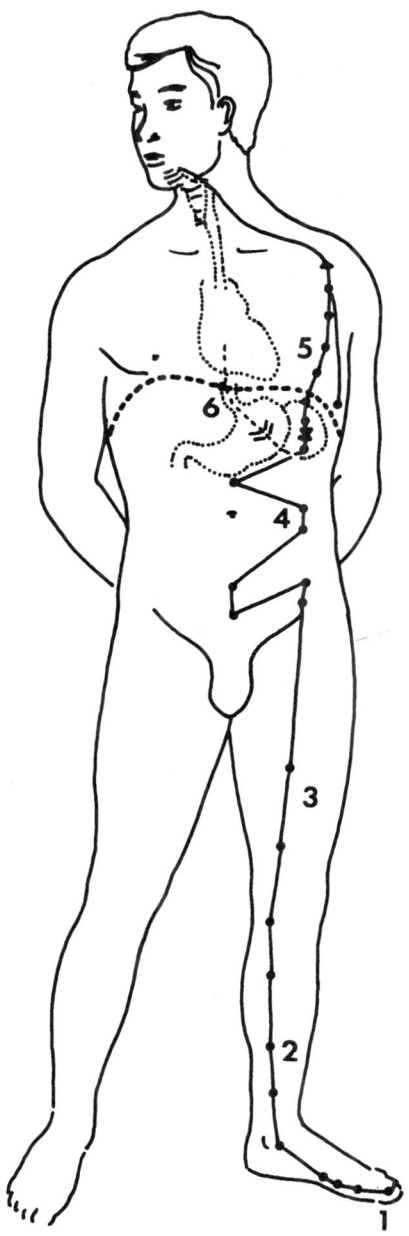

Foot Greater Yin Spleen Channel

(Numbers indicate the direction of the flow of the Qi.)

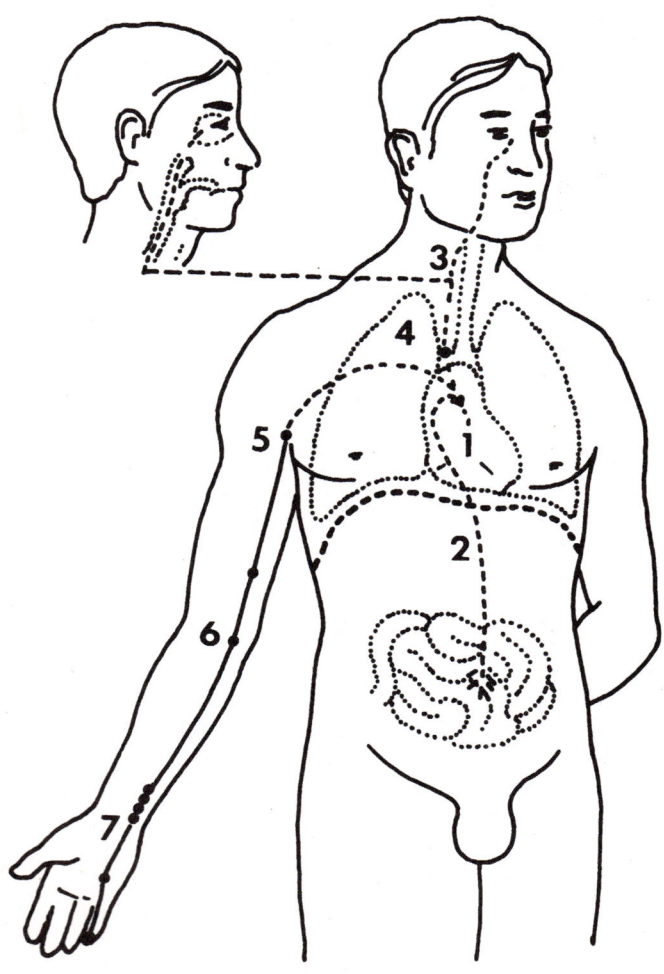

Hand Lesser Yin Heart Channel

(Numbers indicate the direction of the flow of the Qi.)

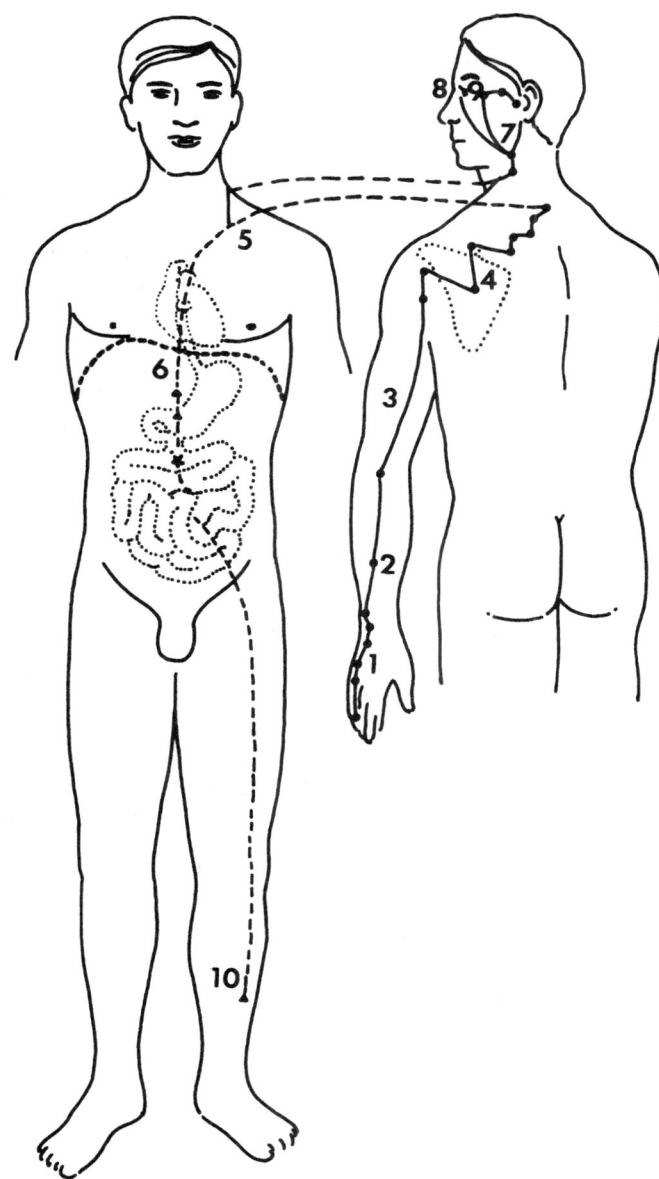

Hand Greater Yang Small Intestine Channel

(Numbers indicate the direction of the flow of the Qi.)

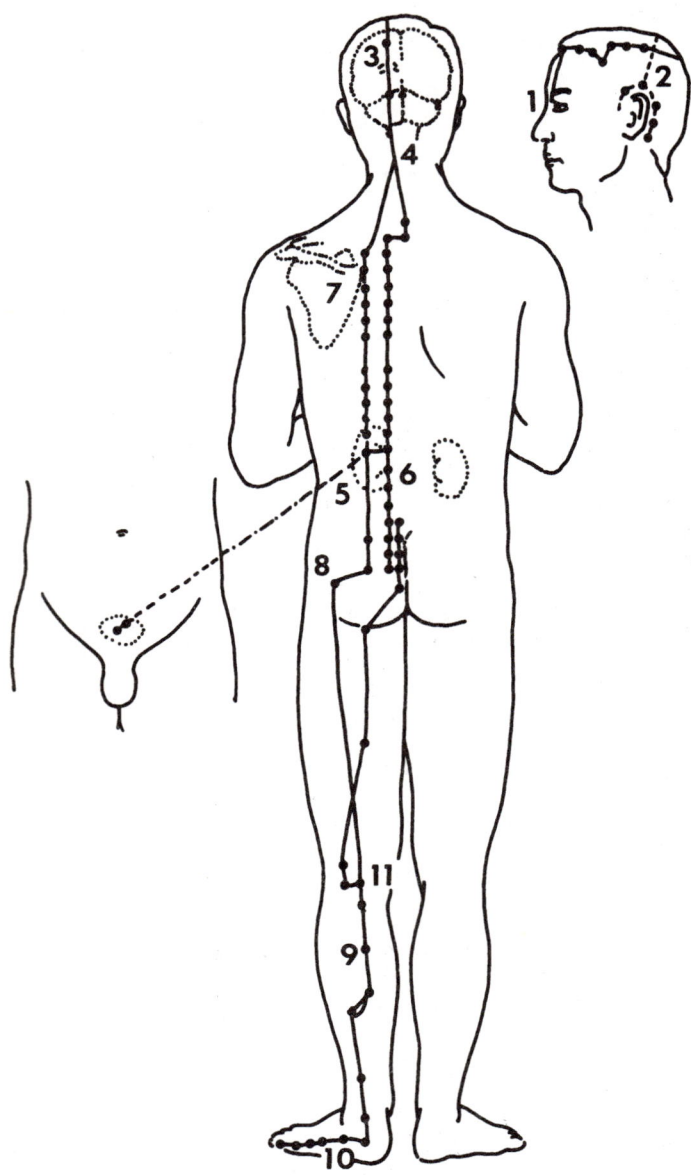

Foot Greater Yang Urinary Bladder Channel

(Numbers indicate the direction of the flow of the Qi.)

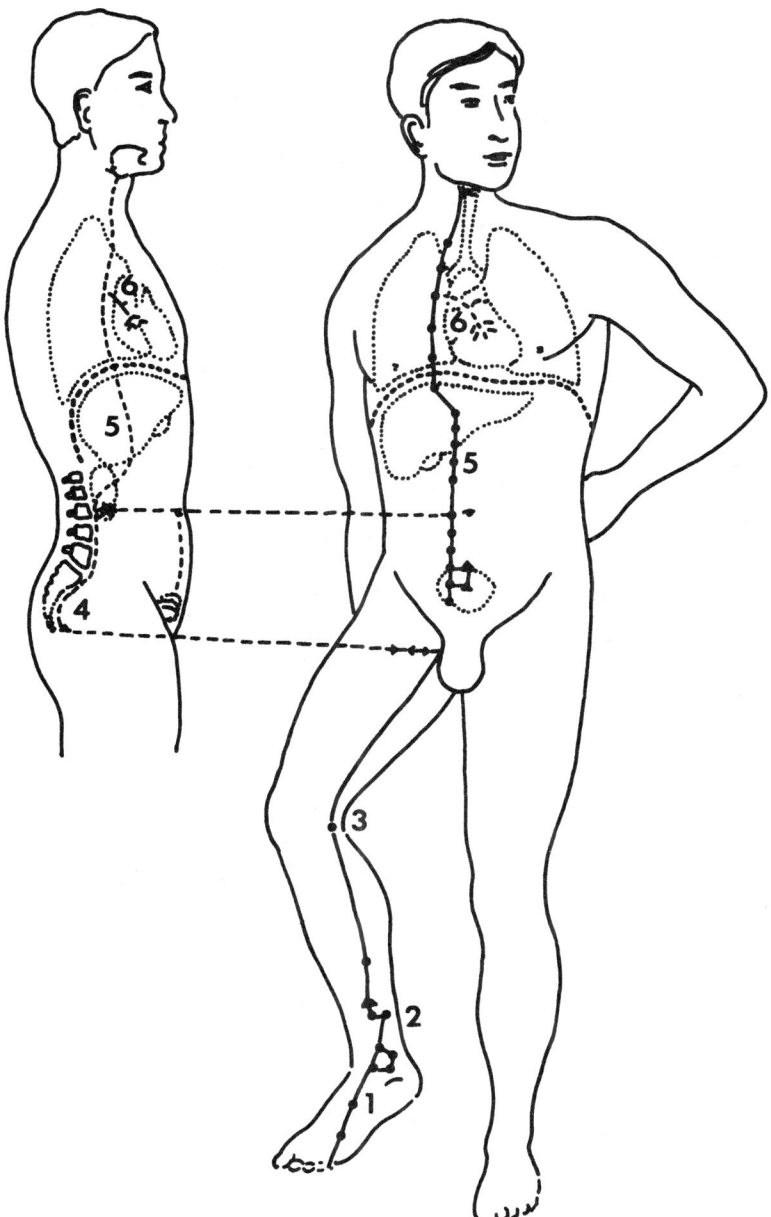

Foot Lesser Yin Kidney Channel

(Numbers indicate the direction of the flow of the Qi.)

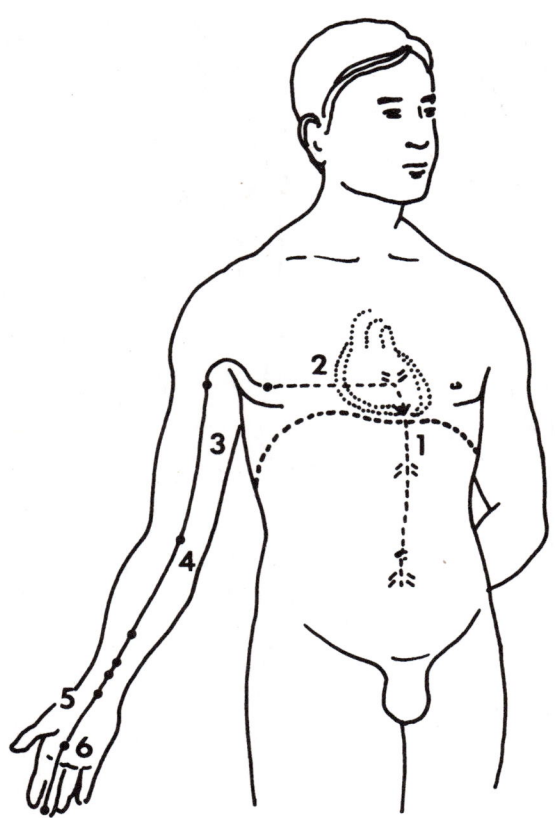

Hand Terminal Yin Pericardium Channel

(Numbers indicate the direction of the flow of the Qi.)

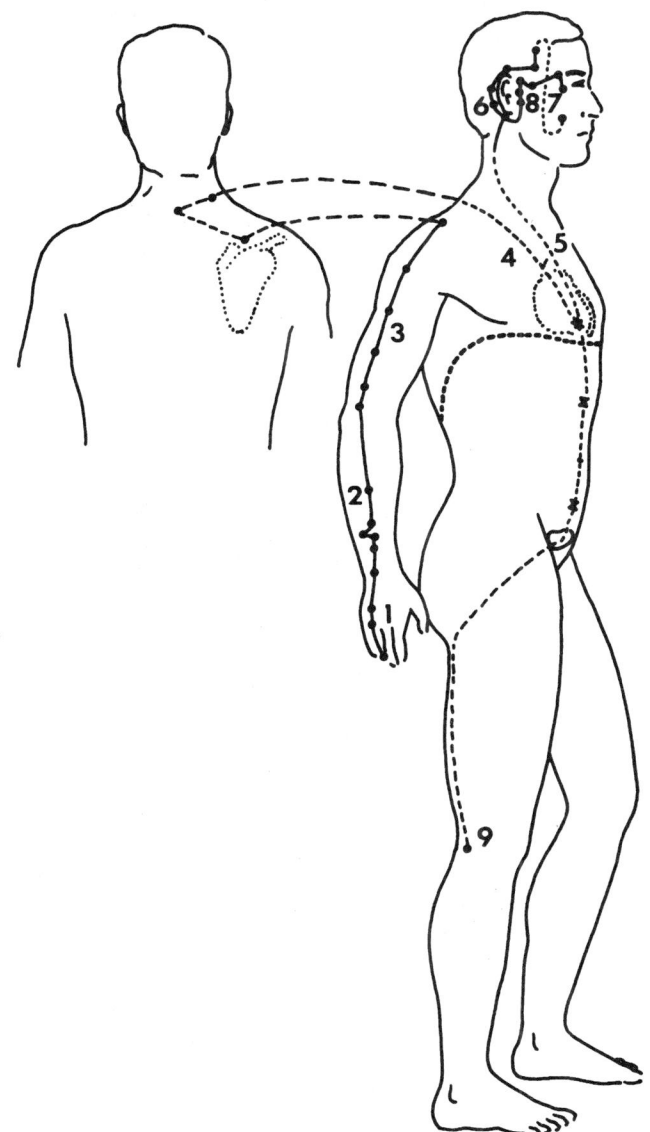

Hand Lesser Yang Triple Energiser Channel

(Numbers indicate the direction of the flow of the Qi.)

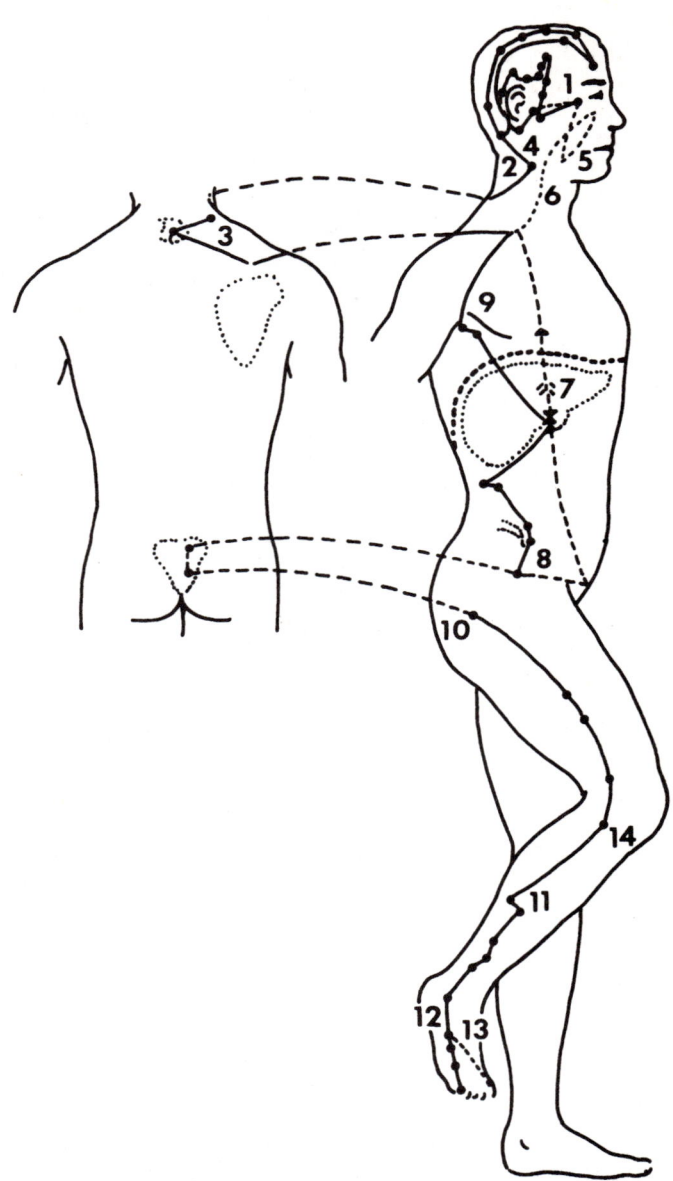

Foot Lesser Gall Bladder Channel

(Numbers indicate the direction of the flow of the Qi.)

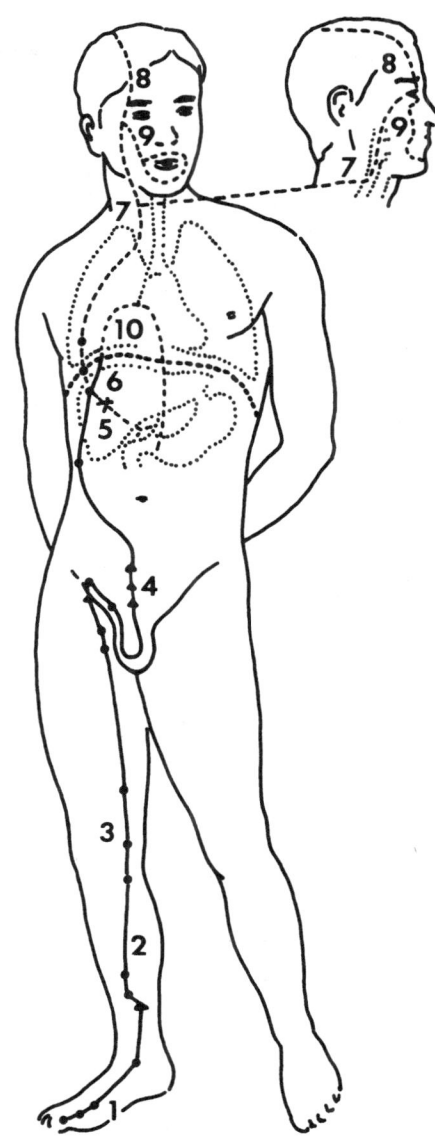

Foot Terminal Yin Liver Channel

(Numbers indicate the direction of the flow of the Qi.)

As for the yang channels, the channel where the yang Qi is beginning to rise is referred to as the Lesser Yang Channels; the one where there is a preponderance of the yang Qi is the Greater Yang Channel; while the channel where the yang Qi reaches the zenith of its flow is referred to as the Bright Yang Channel.

Flowing along the upper extremities are the following three yin channels: the Hand Greater Yin Lung Channel, the Hand Terminal Yin Pericardium Channel and the Hand Lesser Yin Heart Channel. The three yang channels which flow along the upper extremities are the: Hand Bright Yang Larger Intestine Channel, Hand Lesser Yang Triple Energiser Channel and Hand Greater Yang Small Intestine Channel.

Flowing along the lower extremities are the three yin channels: the Foot Lesser Yin Kidney Channel, the Foot Terminal Yin Liver Channel and the Foot Greater Yin Spleen Channel. The three yang channels which flow along the lower extremities are: The Foot Greater Yang Urinary Bladder Channel, the Foot Lesser Yang Gall Bladder Channel, and the Foot Bright Yang Stomach Channel.

The three yin channels along the upper extremities, which emanate from the chest, flow along the inner side of both arms and terminate at the fingers. The yang channels along the upper extremities start from the fingers of both hands and then flow along the outer sides of the arms to terminate at the head and face.

The yang channels along the lower extremities start from the head and face, and then, in separate pathways, flow along either the front, side or back of the trunk down to the outer sides of the lower extremities to terminate at the toes. The yin channels along the lower extremities start from the toes and then flow up along the inner side of the leg to terminate in the abdomen and chest.

Both the yin and yang channels meet in the hand and foot and also there are meeting points of the yang channels in the head while those of the yin channels are in the chest and abdomen. This then constitutes the circulatory network of the 12 regular channels.

The more detailed flow of the Hand Greater Yin Lung Channel is traced and outlined on page 100.

This channel begins from the region of the middle Energiser, which corresponds to the stomach area (1), moves down to the large intestine with which it connects, flows back to and crosses the diaphragm (2), enters the lung organ system with which it is associated, moves up to the throat (3), flows down to the inner side of the shoulder (4), arm and elbow (5), continues to flow down the forearm, passing the area where the radial pulse is taken (6) and then moves towards the tip of the thumb. A branch of this channel splits at the pulse region and diverts towards the tip of the index finger (7) and connects with the Hand Bright Yang Large Intestine Channel which flows towards the body. There are 11 acupoints which dot this channel from the shoulder down to the tip of the thumb, including the acupoint Junction Valley (which will be discussed later).

If this channel is affected by external pathogenic factors or becomes deficient, clinical patterns consisting of signs and symptoms associated with the area of flow along this channel emerge. This clinical pattern would be: coughing, wheezing, chest congestion, distention, shortness of breath, fever, aversion to cold, sweating, pain along the junction of the chest and shoulder, pain along the shoulder, upper back and inner side of the arm, hot sensation in the middle of palm. To address this clinical pattern, acupoints along the Hand Greater Yin Lung Channel and associated channels are needled. (The other channels are the Governor Channel which runs along the mid-spine and the Conception Channel which runs along the midline of the chest and abdomen.)

DIAGNOSING CLINICAL PATTERNS AND ACUPUNCTURE

The choice of acupoints, needling techniques and supplementary procedures all depend upon the presenting clinical pattern of a particular patient. Using the method of differentiating clinical patterns and tailoring treatment principles, a patient's signs and symptoms are assembled into a clinical pattern by using the Four Examination Techniques and then ordered in accordance with the Conceptual Templates of Patterns of Acupuncture Channels (see Chapter I).

In general terms signs and symptoms of coughing, sore throat, wheezing and chest pains could indicate disharmonies affecting the Hand Greater Yin Lung Channel; diarrhoea and lower abdominal pains could indicate disharmonies of the Leg Bright Yang Large Intestine Channel; lower back and back pains could indicate disharmony in the Leg Greater Yang Urinary Bladder Channel or the Leg Greater Yin Kidney Channel and diseases affecting the mouth, nose and face could indicate disharmonies in one of several channel systems.

Once the signs and symptoms of a particular patient have been assembled in accordance with disharmonies reflected in one or more acupuncture channels, then the choice of acupuncture points and related procedures is made.

THE ACUPUNCTURE NEEDLE

There are many types of acupuncture needles. The most commonly used one is called the filiform needle which in Chinese is called 'hao zhen' 毫针. 'Hao' means very minute and fine, similar to a hair strand, and 'zhen' refers to needles in general.

The filiform acupuncture needle is usually made of stainless steel, although there are also silver and gold-plated acupuncture needles. In ancient times, iron acupuncture needles were used; these were thicker and rusted, and they broke easily. The more durable and smoother gold and silver ones were rare and precious.

The part of the acupuncture needle which distinguishes it from other types of needles, such as the syringe needle, is the tip, which is shaped like a pine leaf tip, i.e. sharp but rounded, polished, smooth and straight. The tip should be sharp enough to quickly penetrate the skin and underlying tissues painlessly (although the skills of the acupuncturist are equally relevant). The smoothness and roundness prevents tissue laceration, so that, while a hypodermic needle slices the tissues, an acupuncture needle pushes aside the tissue with minimal damage. The smoothness and roundness also enhances the stimulating effect on nerve receptors embedded in muscular tissues. Ancient Chinese medical literature details that the tip of the acupuncture needle should be shaped like the proboscis of a mosquito or a horsefly, as this shape stabilises the needle's position, keeping it in place when it has been inserted in the skin and underlying tissues. Recent research in China has confirmed that it is the tip of the filiform needle which is responsible for the 'arrival of the Qi' or 'de Qi' (Shen, 1989), the acupuncture sensation which is essential to therapeutic efficacy.

The other parts of the filiform needle are the body, root, handle and tail. The body is that section between the needle tip and the handle, the root is that point which separates the body from the handle, while the tail is the other end of the needle.

The handle is made from silver and copper threads which are coiled around the blunt end of the needle body to form a larger protruding structure which facilitates needle manipulation by the finger and prevents the needle from sinking into the skin tissue.

As for the bodies of acupuncture needles, they vary in length from 13–75 mm, and in diameter or gauge from 0.23–0.45 mm. The fine needles are generally used on sensitive or first-time patients, while thicker needles are appropriate for less sensitive patients and for conditions involving loss of sensory perception, e.g. paralysis resulting from a stroke.

The shorter needles are used for points on the ears, face and fingertips; 25 mm needles are used on the hands, arms, upper back, scalp, neck and chest; 40–50 mm needles may be used on the leg, shoulders, lower back and lower and mid-abdomen; and 75 mm needles may be used for buttocks and thigh points. Even longer needles may be used for overweight patients.

Aside from the filiform needle, there are other types of acupuncture needles such as dermal needles, ear studs, the plum-blossom or seven star needle etc.

ACUPUNCTURE NEEDLING AND MANIPULATION TECHNIQUES

The three basic steps in needling with the filiform needle are insertion, needling motion and withdrawal. There are various techniques of insertion, however the basic requirement is that it be executed quickly and painlessly. Presently plastic tubes are used to facilitate needle insertion and lessen the possibility of cross-infection. Certain acupoints require different methods of needle insertion.

Needling motion or xing zhen 行针 is a technique which involves thrusting the needle inwards and outwards, and rotating the handle clockwise or anti-clockwise once the needle has penetrated the skin. It may also involve flicking or scraping the needle handle up and down with the fingernails. This technique facilitates the arrival of the Qi or de Qi. After the Qi has arrived, the needle is left in place for a period of time. This is called liu zhen 留针. It is not only the patient who feels the arrival of the Qi. When the practitioner manipulates the needle handle and Qi is obtained, she or he can feel a sensation similar to getting a bite on a fishing line. If the Qi is not obtained, it feels as if the needle has been pushed through butter, giving an empty and hollow sensation.

Certain needling techniques used in inserting, moving and withdrawing the needles can achieve tonification to address deficient clinical patterns or sedation to address excess clinical patterns. For example, tonification is achieved when the needle site is pressed with cotton wool immediately after withdrawal. Sedation is achieved when the needle is pulled out slowly and slightly, and simultaneously moved sidewards to widen the point of withdrawal. In such a case, the needle site is not pressed with cotton wool after needle withdrawal.

Another way of achieving tonification is to insert the needle slowly and then withdraw it quickly. The reverse action achieves sedation. Rotating the needle clockwise also brings about tonification, whereas an anti-clockwise action achieves sedation.

Needling can also be combined with the patient's breathing to bring about tonification and sedation. Tonification occurs when the needle is inserted while the patient is exhaling and withdrawn when inhaling. Conversely, sedation occurs when the procedure is reversed. The above are some of the most basic needling techniques which, when combined, form compound needling motion techniques. In total there are approximately 100 simple and compound needling motion techniques.

MOXIBUSTION Jiu 灸

Moxibustion therapy involves the searing or burning of dry herbs and directing this heat to certain acupuncture points. As stated earlier, moxibustion or jiu 灸 constitutes one of the Chinese characters for acupuncture. The use of heat is mainly for cold and deficient clinical patterns, which include signs and symptoms of chills, and the slowing down of the body's metabolism.

The most commonly used herb for moxibustion is mugwort (*Artemisia vulgaris*). The dried and compressed leaves are made into cones and burnt over acupoints until the patient considers the heat unbearable. Sometimes, a slice of garlic or ginger is sandwiched between the moxa cone and the acupoint to address more severe cold patterns.

Specially manufactured cigar-shaped moxa sticks are held a few centimetres away from the acupoints and moved slightly away when the patient feels the heat to be unbearable. They may also be cut into half-inch lengths and placed on the handles of acupuncture needles. Sometimes, longer pieces of moxa stick are placed inside a moxa box and burnt over acupuncture points along the back or abdomen.

Apart from targeting cold and deficient clinical patterns, moxibustion is also used for preventative purposes. Moxibustion on certain acupoints is used to prevent respiratory infections, especially during outbreaks of epidemics.

ELECTRIC ACUPUNCTURE DEVICE *DIAN ZHEN* 电针

Electrical energy is commonly used with acupuncture. In 1953, it became one of the first modern technological developments to successfully integrate with acupuncture and provided the impetus for the breakthrough in acupuncture anaesthesia for surgical purposes.

The most commonly used electrical device is the pulse transistor, which is powered by batteries. It comes in various sizes and with a number of controls to regulate electrical pulse frequencies and intensity. Various types of wavelengths can be produced. The device has several tiny electrical outlets for the wires, which are then clipped to the handles of the acupuncture needles.

Once the needles are inserted into acupoints and the Qi has been obtained, then appropriate needled points are connected to the acupuncture device. The intensity and frequency of the pulse stimulus is set in accordance with the patient's tolerance level for optimum effect. Although duration varies according to the clinical condition, it is generally 10–15 minutes, with a maximum of 30 minutes.

Some devices are fitted with separate outlets, wiring and a point-locating rod. The rod works on the principle that acupoints have low electrical resistance, so they can be detected by running the rod along the surface of the body.

THERAPEUTIC REACTION TO ACUPUNCTURE

When acupuncture is administered properly vis-a-vis the targeted clinical pattern, the patient should respond favourably, so that by the end of the course of treatment, the patient should be free from the signs and symptoms of disease. Comprehensive research in China has confirmed that acupuncture can be therapeutically effective in treating a wide range of diseases affecting all the physiological systems of the body as defined in Western medicine, i.e. digestive, respiratory, musculoskeletal, gynaecological, neurological, psychiatric, urogenital, circulatory, endocrinal etc.

As for individual responses to acupuncture, the experience should be that of obtaining Qi. A radiating sensation which extends towards a definite direction and length can sometimes also be felt. Some sensation at the needle sites may persist for a number of hours after the treatment. After treatment, one should feel relaxed and light in the body. Some patients experience a feeling of 'walking on thin clouds'. If this occurs, do not panic but rest for a while until it passes. Most patients report a good, sound night's sleep. To promote and sustain the therapeutic effects of acupuncture, avoid alcohol before and for two to three hours after the treatment. More importantly, heed the TCM practitioner's advice on how best to deal with your illness.

Below are some of the most commonly used acupoints, their location, therapeutic actions and clinical indications.

Junction Valley He gu 合谷 LI 4

Location: This is the fourth acupoint along the Large Intestine Channel. It is located at the highest point of the bulge of muscle tissue formed when the thumb and index fingers are placed side by side.

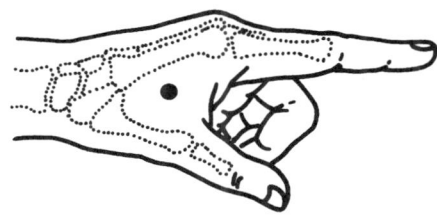

Junction Valley LI 4

Needling Sensation: This is a relatively sensitive point. When needled, a localised tingling and numb sensation, sometimes radiating towards the index finger is felt. The points on both hands are used.

Therapeutic Action: 1. Eliminates heat and releases stagnated Qi along the Large Intestine Channel when a reducing or sedating needling manipulation is used on this point (to deal with an excess clinical pattern).
2. Restores consciousness when strong reduction needling manipulation is applied.
3. Tonifies the Qi when it is deficient.
4. Releases external wind-heat clinical patterns.

Clinical Indications: Commonly used for clinical patterns affecting the head, face, eyes, head and mouth (area to which the Large Intestine Channel flows). It is thus used for conditions like headache and dizziness.

Interior Pass Nei Guan 内关 P 6

Location:	This is the sixth acupoint along the Pericardium Acupuncture Channel. It is about two fingers' breadth above the wrist crease, in between the middle tendons of the forearm.
Acupuncture Sensation:	It is common to experience a radiation sensation, similar to a quick electric current, when this point is needled.
Therapeutic Action:	1. Unblocks the flow of stagnant Qi along the Pericardium Channel when a sedating needling technique is applied.
	2. Calms the spirit, pacifies the stomach and stops vomiting when reducing needling is used on this point.
Clinical Indications:	Insomnia, vomiting, palpitations, asthma and morning sickness.

Three Leg Regulator Zu San Li 足三理 S 36

Location:	This point is located four fingers' breadth down from the outer eye of the knee on the outer upper leg. The name of this point indicates its therapeutic action of regulating the functions of the internal organ systems distributed in the three — upper, middle and lower — regions of the abdominal and chest cavities.
Acupuncture Sensation:	Stimulating this point may produce a localised heavy numb sensation which may sometimes shoot down the front part of the leg to the second smallest toe.
Therapeutic Action:	1. When moxa is applied over this point regularly, it can boost the body's anti-pathogenic Qi and thus prevent illness, keep the body healthy and promote longevity.
	2. When reinforcing or tonifying type of needling or stimulus is applied to this point, it can tonify the spleen system.
	3. Regulates the function of the stomach system and unblocks the intestines, eliminates phlegm and releases stagnated Qi when sedating needling is applied over this point.
Clinical Indications:	Loose bowel motion, constipation, epigastric pains, vomiting, prolapse of the uterus, irregular periods and impotence.

Three Yin Junction San Yin Jiao 三阴交 SP 6

Location:	This is a point three fingers' breadth above the highest point of the inner ankle joint where the three yin channels of the leg (i.e. the spleen, liver and kidney acupuncture channels) converge.
Acupuncture Sensation:	When this point is needled a radiating sensation may be felt similar to a running electric current.
Therapeutic Action:	1. Tonifies the spleen system, thereby tonifying deficient blood when reinforcing or tonifying needling is applied.
	2. When reducing or sedating needling is applied, it can promote blood flow, thereby eliminating blood stasis.
	3. Cools the blood when reducing needling is applied, combined with manipulations to induce cold sensations.
Clinical Indication:	Irregular periods, period pains, abdominal pains after childbirth, infertility, insomnia, forgetfulness, chest pains and bleeding disorder.

Hundred Meetings Bai Hui 百会 GV 20

Location:	This is a point midway between an imaginary line drawn between the apex of both ears on the top of the head. It is the converging point of all the yang acupuncture channels, i.e. the Governing Channel, Large Intestine, Stomach, Small Intestine, Urinary Bladder, Triple Energiser and Gall Bladder Channels, hence the name.
Acupuncture Sensation:	A localised numb sensation may be felt. The acupuncture needle is placed very superficially below the scalp.
Therapeutic Action:	1. When reinforcing or tonifying needling is applied, it tonifies the yang Qi.
	2. Restores the yang when there is loss of consciousness and brings back consciousness when moxa is applied locally.
	3. When reduction needling is applied to this point, it can unblock the Governing Channel, eliminate pathogenic wind and relieve spasms.
Clinical Indications:	Headaches, dizziness, loss of consciousness, physical debility, prolapse of the uterus, epilepsy, diarrhoea, enuresis, sinusitis etc.

Middle Stomach Zhong Wan 中脘 CV 12

Location: This acupoint is midway between the navel and the base of the sternum, hence the name. It is the twelfth acupoint along the Conception Vessel Channel and is the converging point of the six hollow organs and the middle energiser.

Acupuncture Sensation: There is usually only a tiny pinprick of a sensation when the needle goes through the skin and then a slight heavy numbing sensation locally when the needle goes under the skin.

Therapeutic Action:
1. When sedating needling is applied to this acupoint, it can regulate the flow of the stomach Qi and thereby release stagnant Qi along the Stomach Channel, eliminate mucus and dissipate accumulated mass.
2. Tonifies the stomach yang Qi and eliminates cold pathogenic factors when moxibustion is applied.
3. When reinforcing needling is applied, it can tonify the stomach system and the middle energiser.

Clinical Indications: Stomach pains, vomiting, abdominal pains and constipation.

Big Vertebra Da Zhui 大椎 GV 14

Location: This acupoint is located just below the seventh cervical vertebra (the biggest protruding vertebra when the head is bowed), hence the name. It is the meeting point of all the yang acupuncture channels.

Acupuncture Sensation: A localised heavy and sometimes diffused radiating sensation is felt when this point is needled.

Therapeutic Action:
1. When sedating needling is applied over this acupoint it can release exterior clinical patterns and bring down fever.
2. When reinforcing needling is applied over this point it can activate the yang Qi and strengthen the exterior. It is thus used for the prevention of common cold conditions.

Clinical Indications: External clinical patterns, uncontrolled sweating, headache and coughing.

Welcome Fragrance Ying Xiang 迎香 LI 20

Location:	This acupoint is located just slightly above the outer edges of both nostrils. The name comes from the therapeutic function of this point which can unblock the nasal passage and thus restore the sense of smell.
Acupuncture Sensation:	A localised swelling sensation may be felt when this point is needled.
Therapeutic Action:	When sedating needling is applied to this point, it can unblock the nasal passage as well as disperse pathogenic heat.
Clinical Indication:	Acute and chronic rhinitis, allergic rhinitis, sinusitis, trigeminalia and facial muscle spasms.

ADVERSE REACTIONS TO ACUPUNCTURE

When performed properly, acupuncture is a very safe therapeutic discipline. With a long track record of more than two thousand years of use in China, its practice has been continuously improved and refined. However, as with all medical procedures, adverse reactions do occur. Prevention and skilful management of these reactions are essential. Below are some common adverse reactions observed in China and Australia.

Local Haematoma: Minor bleeding sometimes occurs after the needles are withdrawn. Pressing with sterile cotton wool stops the bleeding. Sometimes a slight bruising remains which will eventually disappear after a period of time. A slight haematoma can sometimes later appear on the needle site. When this occurs, apply a warm compress to make it subside.

Fainting or 'needle shock': This can sometimes happen with first-time patients or those who are hungry, lack sleep, nervous, stressed or who have a combination of these factors. The patient turns pale, feels dizzy and then faints. An experienced and alert TCM practitioner should easily notice early signs of fainting and take measures to prevent it.

ACUPUNCTURE-RELATED ACCIDENTS

Acupuncture-related accidents have been reported in China and internationally. In China, while there is university training in TCM and professional registration, the practice of acupuncture in the vast countryside is still in the hands of lesser trained practitioners. Outside of China, while TCM and professional acupuncture organisations are setting standards, there are still no universally recognised training or standards of any sort of TCM, including acupuncture practice. Because of this lack of training and standards, the occurrence of acupuncture-related accidents is always a possibility.

Some of the more serious though rarely occurring accidents include:

- Injury to major internal organs: Poor training in the anatomy of the underlying structures of acupuncture points or poor training in acupuncture needling manipulations, can cause needles to be inserted too deeply, resulting in damage to major internal organs.

- Cross-infection: This is due to the use of dirty and unsterile needles and other instruments. In Australia, most TCM and acupuncture associations advocate the use of disposable needles. This measure, to a large extent, prevents cross-infection.

- Broken needle while the needle is embedded in the skin and subcutaneous tissues. The needle body can break due to muscular contractions of the patient or physical imperfections of the needle or both. This type of accident is rare and most unlikely to occur, especially if disposable needles are used.

A MODERNIST ACCOUNT OF HOW ACUPUNCTURE WORKS

Because of the widespread clinical practice of acupuncture and the impetus provided by the success of acupuncture anaesthesia in China, modern scientific methods have been used to investigate how this ancient system of practice works. In the process, the various ingredients of its practice are being 'translated' from their ancient beginnings into a modern setting. The focus of these research endeavours is on acupuncture sensations (de Qi), acupuncture propagated sensation (gan chuan), the anatomy and physiology of acupuncture points and meridians, and ancient classical literature. (Acupuncture propagated sensations radiate along the acupuncture channel pathways.)

Serious research on all aspects of the practice of acupuncture is at present centred in China. Current research in the West tends to focus only on the biomedical aspects. One school of researchers in China is of the view that the regulatory effects of acupuncture are brought about through its comprehensive effect upon the central nervous and the humoral systems. Specifically, acupuncture stimulus can have a regulatory or therapeutic effect upon the sympathetic nervous, digestive, respiratory, endocrine, cardiovascular, urological, reproductive, immunological, blood and lymphatic systems. However, this regulatory effect is contingent upon the physiological state of the subject, the selection of specific acupoint points, the amount of stimulation, the type of needling technique and the quality of sensation elicited.

A sensation felt during acupuncture is critical to the efficacy of acupuncture therapy. For purposes of analysis, acupuncture sensations or de Qi may be categorised into localised sensations of soreness, distention, heaviness, numbness, radiation and pain. Depending upon which of the 2000 acupuncture points are stimulated by the needle, the sensation is a composite sensory perception which may be a blending or accentuation of one or several of these sensations.

Research conducted in China confirms that acupuncture sensation results from the fine acupuncture needle's smooth tip touching the skin and layers of tissues underneath. The real chance to validate the anatomical basis of acupuncture sensations came with the development of acupuncture anaesthesia in the 1970s, when surgery was performed on conscious patients. During these operations layers of tissues (from the skin to the bone), which correspond to particular acupoints, were stimulated and the patient's responses recorded.

The studies revealed that when the needle stimulates nerve fibres it elicits numbness; when it touches the blood vessels it elicits pain; when it touches the periosteum (the surrounding tissue of the bone) and tendons it elicits soreness and when it touches muscle it elicits sensations of distention and soreness. Subsequent studies confirmed that the structural and physical source of acupuncture sensations are deep nerve receptors underneath acupuncture points.

Concentrations of nerve receptors called neuromuscular spindles were found under acupoints abundant in muscular tissues, such as Zu San Li (S 36) and under acupoints where muscular tissues and tendons converge, such as Chang Shan (B 57). Receptors in the form of free nerve endings were found in tissues under specific acupoints located on the scalp and face, such as Bai Hui (GV 20). Receptors called Pacini's corpuscles were found in tissues underneath acupoints located along tendons, e.g. Kun Lun (B 60). Nerve receptors called Ruffini's corpuscles were found underneath the acupoint Du Bi (S 35) inside the knee joint capsule.

Acupuncture Nerve Pathway

As a result of research on acupuncture anaesthesia, the specific CNS (central nervous system) pathway along which the acupuncture impulses run is also becoming better understood, and the specific centres in the brain which participate in the mechanisms of acupuncture are becoming defined.

It is now clear that from the nerve receptors underneath acupoints, the information signal is relayed to the dorsal horn neurons of the spinal cord. At this level, through a segmental circuit, the acupuncture information signal reacts on the lateral or ventral horn neurons of the spinal cord. There it influences any initial integration of the pain stimulus.

The information signal then ascends to the higher centres of the brain through the ventro-lateral cell column of the spinal cord. First it goes to the centres within the brain stem, known as the reticular formation and the median raphe, where further integration occurs between the acupuncture information signal and the pain stimulus. From the brain stem, the acupuncture information signal ascends to the thalamus, the central nucleus of the brain, where it triggers an inhibitory impulse that dampens the activities of the pain-sensitive neurons of the thalamus.

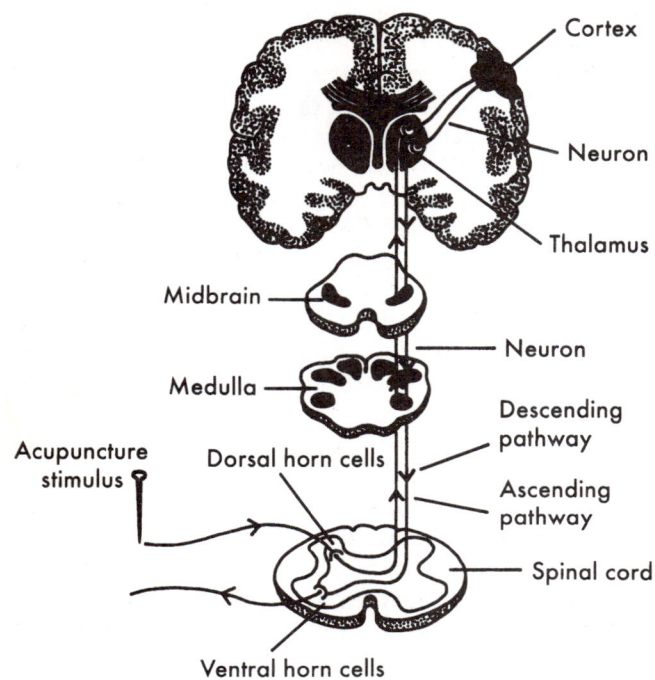

Acupuncture Nerve Pathway

From the thalamus, the information signal descends again to the brain stem, travels further down the dorsal lateral column to the spinal cord's dorsal horn neurons. Here, this descending impulse exerts a powerful control over any incoming pain signal. It also regulates the activities of the sympathetic nerve fibre (part of the body's self-regulatory, non-voluntary nervous system), which operates as the efferent nerve.

Acupuncture Nerve Circuit

A cycle is thus established where an acupuncture signal affects the nervous system's perception of pain both in the spinal cord and the brain, and also affects the body's organs directly.

As an example, needling the bilateral acupoints Zu San Li (S 36), on the upper frontal region of the shin bone, decreases peristaltic movement of the stomach. In this case, the stimulus travels from the shin up the peroneal nerve to the CNS, where integration with the pain signal takes place.

Information is sent back along the sympathetic nerves to the stomach, reducing intestinal activity. Furthermore, the effects of acupuncture do not end with the withdrawal of the stimulus. Usually, if the treatment is applied properly, the treatment lasts for an extended period of time. This phenomenon is due to changes in endocrine or glandular secretions accompanying the CNS effects of the acupuncture stimulus.

It has also been confirmed that acupuncture increases the level of endorphins (naturally occurring narcotic hormones) in the blood which enhance the analgesic effects of acupuncture.

Acupuncture's Role in Maintaining the Body's Equilibrium

Based upon the phenomenon of the arrival of Qi, as well as the sensation which radiates or propagates from the acupoints, which corresponds to the ancient channel circuit, another group of researchers in China theorised that the channel system is one of the four physiological systems in the body which maintains equilibrium (Meng, 1983). The other three systems are: the somatic nervous system, the sympathetic nervous system and the endocrine or glandular system.

The somatic nervous system maintains rapid posture equilibrium; the sympathetic nervous system maintains equilibrium in the functioning of the internal organs; and the endocrine system maintains slow equilibrium for the whole of the body's physiological functions. The acupuncture channel system, it was suggested, maintains equilibrium between the surface of the body and the internal organs by decreasing an over-active bodily function or activating a depressed one. These four systems together may be compared to stabilisers in a complicated piece of electronic equipment or a brake mechanism in a motor car.

In differentiating these four systems, the speed of response-to-stimuli conduction was measured and compared. In the case of the somatic nerves, the speed of conduction is 100 metres per second; the speed of conduction in the sympathetic nerve system is one metre per second; and the speed in the endocrine system was measured in terms of minutes. In the case of acupuncture's needling technique, the speed of response-to-stimuli conduction was 10 centimetres per second. The researchers noted the big gap between the sympathetic and endocrine systems which led them to conclude that the acupuncture channel system seems to fill this gap.

For a period of six years, the acupuncture channel networks were studied, using 100 acupuncture channel-sensitive people (people who record physical reactions like lines of skin blemishes or feel sensations which radiate along the acupuncture pathways). Traditional methods of acupuncture were used.

Comparing these studies with descriptions of the channel networks in the ancient texts, the researchers discovered interesting similarities and differences. For example, they discovered that all channels travel towards the head, as opposed to the ancient channel description and illustrations, which show that the yin channels do not flow towards the head.

Also, while the flow of all 12 channels demonstrate striking similarities to the ancient illustrations when they flow along the extremities, they show great disparities when they flow towards the body and the head. Modern research also showed that the Foot Greater Yang Urinary Bladder Channel, which runs along the back, links up with the other 11 channels. This, too, differs significantly from the ancient illustrations and descriptions.

• C H A P T E R   V I I •

TUINA: CHINESE THERAPEUTIC MASSAGE

推拿

'TUINA' IS THE CHINESE TERM FOR THERAPEUTIC MASSAGE WHICH IS MADE UP OF two Chinese characters, i.e. 'tui' 推 which means to execute a pushing motion with the fingers or hand; and 'na' 拿 which means to grasp with the hand or finger.

Some Chinese historians claim that the word 'massage' originated from an ancient Chinese word 'masa' 摩挲 which means to stroke gently. It is claimed that it was from this Chinese colloquial term used during the Han Dynasty (206 BC–AD 24) that the French word for massage 'masser' evolved when tuina reached France a thousand years ago. Eventually 'masser' became 'massage' in English. Another commonly used Chinese name for therapeutic massage is 'an mo' 按摩. 'An' 按 means to press, while 'mo' 摩 means to rub.

Tuina (which can be pronounced as 'twey nar') is a form of stimulation of varying intensity, direction, frequency and duration applied to specific sites on the surface of the body, i.e. acupoints or channel sites. It involves the rhythmical motions of the fingers, palm, knuckles, elbow and feet tailored to address specific clinical patterns of disharmony. It also involves the use of massage paraphernalia and media, such as oils and essences, to enhance its therapeutic effects.

Tuina is one of the oldest TCM disciplines, having evolved much earlier than acupuncture. Chinese historians surmised that tuina gradually evolved from the primitive experience of accidentally rubbing or pressing certain injured parts of the body and discovering that certain discomfort or conditions were thereby relieved. This experience gradually evolved into a system which identified particular rubbing, pressing or pushing techniques with the alleviation of certain clinical signs and symptoms. The development of philosophical thought in later dynasties gave impetus to the systematisation of this body of knowledge and experience. Eventually specialist books on tuina were written and compiled and handed down from generation to generation.

While there are some basic principles in the practice of tuina, there are also various schools of tuina which reflect different styles of massage technique. Schools may put emphasis on the use of certain techniques, or degrees of intensity, or certain acupoints or certain channels. For example, one school of tuina mainly uses percussion tuina techniques involving a couple of fingers targeted on certain acupoints. Variations are also regional in nature. For example, the Shanghai, Beijing, or Sichuan style of tuina each have distinguishing features. The northern China style of tuina is generally heavy in intensity while the southern style is light.

GENERAL TUINA TECHNIQUES SHOU FA 手法

While the individual herb is the key element in herbal medicine and the acupuncture needle is the key therapeutic device in acupuncture, the various tuina techniques or shou fa are the key to the practice of tuina. In the course of their evolution, massage techniques in China have undergone a long history of systematisation and standardisation, the process of which has been meticulously recorded in ancient and contemporary literature.

Basic and Compound Tuina Techniques

Tuina techniques are classified as basic or compound. There are approximately 20 basic tuina massage techniques, the most common of which are the push, press, grasp, pinch, knead, roll, pluck and dig techniques. Each basic technique has a general therapeutic attribute. These basic techniques are then further classified into compound tuina techniques depending upon which parts of the body are used to execute them (e.g. hands or fingers), the massage direction, its depth, its intensity, and how these techniques are combined with each other.

Push Technique *Tui* 推

This technique involves using the fingers or palm to push up, down or sidewards on the surface of the body. It is generally effective for removing obstruction along the channels and facilitaing Qi circulation. It is particularly beneficial to the heart system. Under this basic categorisation, there are various types of compound push techniques, e.g. straight finger push technique; palm straight push technique; divergent finger push technique; convergent push technique.

Press Technique *An* 按

This involves using the fingers, palms, elbows or feet to apply graduated pressure over certain acupoints or regions of the body. This technique is suitable for alleviating pain in deep tissues, e.g. the bones. It is beneficial for the kidney system and can generally alleviate pain and tonify blood by facilitating Qi flow. Compound press techniques include touch press technique, extended press technique, bent finger press technique and foot treading technique.

Grasp Technique *Na* 拿

This technique involves using the fingers or palms to grasp muscle tissues or tendons of certain acupoints. It massages the muscular tissues and is beneficial for the spleen system. The technique dissipates accumulated heat in certain organ systems and so addresses hot clinical patterns. Compound grasp techniques include: fixed grasp technique, grasp-lifting technique and grasp-pulling technique.

Rub Technique *Mo* 摩

This involves using the fingerpads or palms to lightly apply a circular rubbing motion over certain acupoints. It is generally good for the skin and benefits the lung system. This method can calm the spirit (giving a relaxing effect), alleviate pain and relieve stagnant Qi. Compound rubbing techniques include combing, horizontal, slanting and binding rubs.

Knead Technique *Rou* 揉

This involves using the fingers or palms to apply a slightly heavier circular rubbing massage over certain acupoints. When rubbing, the tissues underneath must sway with the motion of the hand. This technique can enliven blood flow, thereby dispelling stagnation of blood while softening accumulated mass and alleviating pain. Compound kneading techniques include finger kneading, palm kneading and rolling kneading.

Pluck Technique *Bo* 拨

This involves using the thumb and fingers of one hand to pluck the tendon sections of muscular tissues in a similar way to plucking guitar strings. It is generally used for deep tendons and is beneficial to the liver system.

Pinch Technique *Nie* 捏

This involves pinching or squeezing certain muscles or ligaments over certain acupoints to faciliate Qi and blood flow along the channnel and to enliven the spirit. Compound pinching techniques include single-handed pinching and two-handed pinching.

Dig Technique *Qia* 掐

This involves using the fingertips to dig deep and exert pressure over certain acupoints. This technique is applied until the patient feels the de Qi or acupuncture sensation. This method is also referred to as the 'finger needling method' and 'acupressure' because it is similar to acupuncture. Its therapeutic attribute then is contingent upon the acupuncture point on which it is being applied. An example of a compound digging technique is the dig kneading technique.

INDIVIDUAL TUINA TECHNIQUES

Basic and compound tuina techniques are used to stimulate certain acupoints and channels. In the course of tuina evolution, certain combinations or formulae of basic and compound tuina techniques were found to be very effective in dealing with specific clinical patterns. For example, the application of the pinch technique on acupoints Junction Valley (on both hands) was found to be effective in dealing with clinical patterns involving the Hand Greater Yang Large Intestine Channel, i.e. disease affecting the front of the head, mouth, teeth and nasal region.

As a consequence, the therapeutic effects of individual techniques on certain acupoints or channel networks were defined. Over 200 of these have been developed and their therapeutic attributes differentiated. In general terms, individual tuina techniques can have a combination of diaphoretic, tonifying, warming, mediating, clearing, downward draining or emetic effects. Below are examples of individual tuina techniques, their application to certain acupoints and their therapeutic attributes.

Pinch Massage To Junction Valley

Procedure: Place the thumb tip on acupoint Yang Ditch (LI I5), located on the radial (pulse) side of the wrist. Push massage repeatedly with the thumb, towards acupoint Junction Valley (LI 14), i.e. the junction between the first and second metacarpal bones. Continue to the tip of the index finger where the acupoint Shang Yang (LI 1) is located. Massage each hand repeatedly for one to two minutes, after which apply a pinch and dig massage to Junction Valley for two to three minutes.

Therapeutic Action: Dispels pathogenic wind from the exterior of the body and is used to address external clinical patterns. It can also restore consciousness.

Clinical Indications: In conjunction with other individual tuina techniques, it can be used for a wind-cold type external clinical pattern characterised by a runny nose, blocked nostrils, aversion to cold and a superficial pulse. It can also be used for headaches, dizziness, facial paralysis, as well as fainting and loss of consciousness.

Converging Press Massage to Interior Pass (P 6) and Exterior Pass (TE 5)

Procedure: With the thumb on acupoint Great Mound (P 7) on the palmar side of the patient's wrist, and the fingers on acupoint Yang Pool (TE 4) on the dorsal side of the wrist, knead massage repeatedly to the tip of the middle finger for one to two minutes. Place separately the tip of the thumb and index finger on acupoints Internal Pass (P 6) on the palmar side of the forearm and Exterior Pass (TE 5) on the back of the forearm. Apply a converging press massage for three minutes. Localised sensations of soreness and distention will be felt on these acupoints.

Therapeutic Action: Regulates the functioning of the stomach system, calms the spirit and stops pain.

Clinical Indications: In combination with other individual tuina techniques, this can be used for the clinical patterns of stomach system disharmonies with signs and symptoms of stomach pains, nausea and vomiting, and for clinical patterns involving disharmonies of the heart or pericardium systems with signs and symptoms of chest congestion, hurried breathing, palpitations, as well as insomnia and excessive dreams.

Knead Massage To Three Leg Regulator (S 36)

Procedure: Use the protrusion of the back of a bent index finger to apply finger knead massage over the acupoint Three Leg Regulator (S 36) for two to three minutes. Place the four fingers of one hand on acupoint Yang Hill Spring (G 34) on the outer part of the leg and repeatedly stroke-rub massage downwards to the acupoint Hanging Bell (G 39) for one to two minutes. During the application of this tuina technique, localised soreness and distention, as well as a descending, flowing sensation, may be felt.

Therapeutic Action: Regulates the flow of Qi and blood, tonifies the stomach and spleen systems.

Clinical Indications: In conjunction with other individual massage techniques, this technique can deal with disharmonies of stomach and large intestine systems, with symptoms and signs of stomach pains, abdominal distention, intestinal sounds and loss of appetite. It can also be used for signs and symptoms associated with hemiplegia.

Press Massage To Mid-Abdomen

Procedure: The thumb or fingers of one hand are placed on acupoint Upper Stomach (CV 13). From this point apply contact, press massage downwards along the mid-abdomen to Crooked Bone (CV 2) just above the pubic bone, passing through such acupoints as Middle Stomach (CV 12), Lower Stomach (CV 10), Stone Door (CV 5), Sea of Qi (CV 6) and Primordial Qi Storehouse (CV 4). Massage repeatedly 5–10 minutes. The choice of acupoints depends upon the presenting clinical pattern.

Therapeutic Action: Tonifies the spleen and stomach systems, warms the kidney system and strengthens the yang Qi.

Clinical Indications: This technique can be used for a kidney system deficiency with signs and symptoms of irregular periods, post-partum abdominal pains, dysmenorrhoea, impotency, seminal emissions or premature ejaculation.

Knead Massage from Big Vertebra (GV 14) Down To Lower Back Yang Pass (GV 3)

Procedure: Use thumb to apply knead massage to Big Vertebra (GV 14) one to three minutes, after which finger knead massage is applied to Lower Back Yang Pass (GV 3) on the lower back. Apply palm circular kneading massage on these two points for three to five minutes.

Therapeutic Action: Dispels wind and cold pathogenic factors, warms and tonifies the spleen and kidney systems.

Clinical Indications: In conjunction with other tuina techniques, this technique is suitable for a wind-cold external clinical pattern. It can also be used for chest pains, palpitations, shoulder pains and numbness on the upper extremities.

Facial Rub Dig Massage

Procedure: Use thumbs to finger dig massage acupoints Welcome Fragrance (LI 20) on both sides of the nostrils. Then, use thumbs to finger rub massage along the upper jaw bone, moving through acupoints Cheek Seam (SI 18), Lower Pass (S 27) and Ear Door (TE 21) as you progress. Massage repeatedly for one to three minutes.

Therapeutic Action: Enlivens Qi and blood flow along the Large Intestine Channel and stops pain, dispels pathogenic wind and restores consciousness.

Clinical Indications: Used to deal with wind-cold external clinical patterns with symptoms of headache and blocked nose. This technique can also be used for facial paralysis.

REQUIREMENTS FOR TUINA APPLICATION

In general, there are five requirements for applying tuina massage techniques. They should be prolonged, have sufficient strength, be applied evenly, be gentle and achieve penetrating effects.

'Prolonged' means that the tuina technique must be employed for a specified amount of time, usually a couple of minutes or 50 to 100 strokes for each technique. However, the duration can vary with the patient's condition. 'Sufficient strength' in tuina means that the intensity of every technique used is contingent upon the physical constitution of the patient, the illness, the clinical pattern and the site or point massaged. Generally speaking, young, physically robust patients with a strong body constitution can endure a heavier tuina, while children, the elderly and those with weak body constitutions should be given a more moderate and lighter tuina.

A rhythmic flow must be maintained in tuina. It must be light at the beginning, gradually become intense, then heavy, and then as the tuina draws to an end, become lighter and less intense. This is what is meant by 'evenly'. In addition, the speed, direction and intensity must also be evenly applied. 'Gentleness' means that it 'should not be too light like floating in thin air nor too heavy like wallowing in sticky mud'.

'Penetrating effect' refers to the general and localised sensation a patient feels when having tuina. Generally, a correct application of tuina should produce a relaxed and pleasant feeling in the patient. Locally, a warm and loosening sensation may be felt. However for heavy tuina techniques, like the digging technique, a localised de Qi sensation may be felt.

A TUINA FORMULA FOR COMMON COLD

As in acupuncture, tuina exerts its effect upon the acupoint and channel network. To treat clinical conditions, the clinical pattern must first be established so that the appropriate combination or formula of tuina techniques can be tailored for the patient. In establishing this pattern, the practitioner commonly uses the TCM conceptual templates (see page 14), e.g. The Eight Principal Patterns and The Patterns of Acupuncture Channels, to order the signs and symptoms of a patient. Below is an example of how tuina is used to deal with the clinical pattern of a common cold.

The common cold in Chinese is referred to as 'gan mao' 感冒 which means being exposed to or afflicted by extreme weather changes of wind or cold. According to TCM, the common cold is caused by a sudden attack by the pathogenic Qi of wind on the surface of the body, when the anti-pathogenic Qi of the body is weakened. This then causes the lung system to lose its normal physiological function of promoting the flow of Qi to all parts of the body. The lung system extends to the nose and throat and connects with the superficial parts of the body by way of the channel system. Hence, external pathogenic factors like cold wind can affect the lung system through the body's surface.

In accordance with the nature of the pathogenic Qi and the body's response to it, signs and symptoms of the common cold can be differentiated into wind-cold external patterns or wind-heat external patterns. The common signs and symptoms of a wind-heat external pattern are: fever, headache, no sweat, aversion to cold, runny nose, thin-whitish tongue coating, and a superficial and tight pulse.

With the wind-heat external clinical pattern, the therapeutic principle followed is to dispel wind and heat from the exterior. Dispelling wind heat has the effect of sedating or reducing the excess pathogenic factors. The tuina prescriptions used are the following:

a. Rub and dig massage to the face
b. Divergent push massage to the forehead
c. Knead massage from Big Vertebra (GV 14) to Lower Back Yang Pass (GV 3)
d. Grasp lift-massage of the spine
e. Pinch massage to Junction Valley (LI 14).

If the anti-pathogenic Qi needs to be boosted, knead massage to Three Leg Regulator (S 36) may be added.

Normally, the sequence in the use of the above techniques will be given from head to toe and from left to right and back to front. The use of an aromatic massage medium, such as massage oil with peppermint or eucalyptus, is advisable as this can help to dispel pathogenic factors from the exterior.

TUINA EQUIPMENT

Throughout the course of tuina history various equipment has been developed to specifically increase the intensity of stimulus compared with that generated by manual tuina techniques. These aids come in various shapes and sizes depending upon which type of tuina technique they are patterned upon.

Pressure Needle — This metallic instrument, about 7.5–10 cm long, has a tip fashioned like a millet grain. This is mostly used to apply digging tuina techniques on acupoints on the fingers and toes without pricking the skin. Sometimes it is made with a metal encasement with a spring inside to regulate the pressure exerted by the pressure needle.

Round Needle — This metallic tuina apparatus which is shaped like bamboo, is 5–7.5 cm long and less than one centimetre wide, with a rounded tip at both ends. It is used to apply tuina pressure and digging techniques on acupoints located on thicker muscular tissues like the back, arms and neck.

T-Shape Tuina Apparatus — This wooden apparatus, with a handle-like body and a blunt head shaped like a ball, is used to apply a press massage or a pluck tendons massage. It is suitable for areas of the body abundant in muscular tissues, and on patients who are not very sensitive. The apparatus is pressed onto an acupuncture point until the patient feels localised soreness, distention and numbness.

Pistol-Shape Tuina Apparatus — This tuina apparatus is shaped like a pistol and is made of wood or hard plastic. It has a pistol handle and body, and a barrel which is smooth and rounded. The use is similar to the T-shaped tuina apparatus but, since only one hand is used with this device, the pressure exerted is less.

Tuina Crutch — This is a wooden or plastic apparatus in the shape of a crutch, with a crutch handle and body, and a tip which is like a smooth ball. The practitioner puts the crutch handle under his armpit and then places the tip over certain parts of the body to apply pressure. The use is similar to the T-shape tuina apparatus.

Clam Shell Tuina Apparatus — This is a wooden apparatus made in the shape of a clam shell, with a clam body and edge. The practitioner uses part of the shell to apply rubbing, pushing, kneading and plucking tuina massage techniques on the surface of the body. It can be used on the head, neck, extremities and trunk.

Sika Deer Horn — This is the horn of the Sika deer itself, composed of the deer horn root, body and tip. The practitioner holds the horn root and uses the horn tip to apply kneading, plucking, pressing and pushing tuina techniques over certain points on the body. This apparatus is used with the patient's clothes on (which should not be too thick), to protect the skin from possible injury.

Tuina Wheel — This has a round metallic body with ball bearings to make it roll like a wheel, and wooden side handles. The tuina wheel can be used to roll over certain areas of the body. The pressure while rolling the wheel can reach deep into muscular tissues until the patient feels a warm, sore and distended localised feeling. It can be used on the lower back, sacral area, back and lower extremities.

TUINA MEDIA: OIL AND ESSENCES

Traditionally certain massage media are used in tuina. In some cases oil is used as lubrication to prevent injury to the skin resulting from the repeated use of pushing types of tuina techniques. In this respect, it is also worthwhile pointing out that in northern China a piece of cotton cloth of medium thickness is used to protect the skin. The choice of a particular massage medium in tuina is based upon its ability to enhance therapeutic action. In this respect the 'inclinations' or therapeutic attributes of these substances are used to attain this end. The most commonly used massage media in China are ginger juice, egg white, talcum powder, herbal oils, salve and certain strong liquors.

However, in most Western countries the most commonly used massage media are aromatherapy essences mixed with a massage oil base, for example soya bean oil. The therapeutic attributes or 'inclinations' of these herbal essences, as defined in accordance with TCM herbal principles, can enhance the therapeutic attributes of tuina techniques. The most useful oils are euca-lyptus, peppermint and lemongrass.

WHEN NOT TO USE TUINA

Tuina should not be given to patients who have the following conditions:

1. Infectious diseases of the bones, muscular tissues, tendons or joints.
2. Various forms of skin diseases, especially infectious ones.
3. Malignant tumours or cancer.
4. Active bleeding conditions.
5. Dislocated joints.
6. Pregnancy and heavy menstrual bleeding. It is not advisable to apply tuina on the abdominal area or lower back region of pregnant women nor to give a vigorous tuina to a patient having heavy menstrual bleeding at the time.
7. Hunger or a full stomach. Tuina should be administered half an hour before a meal or one and a half hours after a meal.
8. Extreme fatigue.

CHINESE INFANT MASSAGE *Xiao Er Tuina* 小儿推拿

Chinese infant massage is a specialised tuina which emerged during the Ming Dynasty (1368–1644), making it one of the youngest TCM therapeutic disci-plines. It is normally given to babies and children. The points or areas massaged differ significantly from those for adults due to children's immature develop-ment. There are two types of points used for Chinese infant massage: the chan-nel acupoints whose location are similar to those of adults; and special infant massage points. Most of the special infant massage points are located along the arms and hands but are not linked together into a channel network.

The most common tuina massage techniques of pushing, kneading, digging and rubbing etc are also used to massage these points. Giving tuina massage to babies requires special skills, sensitivity and dedication.

Chinese infant massage is effective for the treatment of common paediatric complaints, e.g. repeated colds, diarrhoea, asthma, indigestion, cough, colic, allergy conditions and bed-wetting.

HOW DOES TUINA WORK?

The therapeutic effects of tuina are contingent upon the presenting clinical pattern; the intensity, duration, direction, frequency and intensity of tuina technique applied; and the acupuncture point or channel network used.

Depending upon their yin or yang categorisation, tuina massage techniques may have a sedating or tonifying effect to address yin or yang as well as deficient or excess clinical patterns. Techniques which are applied heavily, deeply or for a protracted period of time are yang types and have a sedating or reducing effect, so these are used for excess clinical patterns. On the other hand, light, shallow, less intense massage techniques applied for a shorter period of time are yin types and generally have a tonifying or reinforcing effect so they can be used to address deficient clinical patterns.

Research from China confirms the neurological basis for the tonifying and sedating effects of tuina. Generally speaking, stimuli from tuina massage techniques which have a short duration, superficial effect and an excitory effect on muscular cellular tissues have a tonifying effect. However, stimuli which have a longer duration, a deep-tissue effect and produce an inhibitory effect upon the muscular cellular tissues have a sedating effect.

Our skin has two types of sensory nerve receptors: excitory effector nerves and inhibiting effector nerves. The excitory nerves are distributed on the superficial layers of the skin and receive the stimulus of touch. The inhibitory effector nerves are concentrated in the deeper layers of the skin and receive pressure stimulus. The excitory effector nerves have premature and early adaptability to stimulus and are referred to as 'rapidly-adapting receptors', while the inhibitory effector nerves have a slow adaptability to stimulus and are hence referred to as 'slow-adapting receptors'. Rapidly-adapting receptor promote or excite muscular activity, while slow-adapting receptors inhibit muscular activity.

When using tuina for the treatment of certain clinical conditions, deep tuina techniques can inhibit hyperactive functions, e.g. local areas on the surface of the body with muscular tension. Deep tuina techniques are not necessarily heavy stimuli, nor are superficial tuina techniques necessarily light stimuli. For example, a stimulus of pressure may be quite deep but not necessarily heavy. On the other hand, a percussion tuina technique may be very heavy but its stimulus felt quite superficially. Stimuli are related to the duration, nature and quality of the tuina massage techniques, so that techniques applied for a protracted period of time do produce a deep stimulus, while those applied for a shorter duration may produce only a superficial stimulus.

As for the therapeutic effects of tuina massage techniques on the physiological functioning of the internal organs of the body, weak and light tuina stimuli can excite physiological functions, while strong tuina massage stimuli can inhibit physiological functions. For example, the use of strong press and contact press tuina massage techniques on acupoints on the back (Stomach Acupoint B 21) in short durations can alleviate stomach or intestinal spasms. Light and protracted push and rub tuina techniques applied on acupoints on the abdomen and back can bring down blood pressure in patients with a 'dampness and phlegm blocking the channel' clinical pattern.

Hence, tuina techniques which produce a strong stimulus in short duration can inhibit physiological activity and so bring about a 'sedating effect', while tuina techniques which produce a light stimulus over a protracted period of time can excite and promote internal organ physiological activity and bring about a tonifying effect. However, the tonifying and sedating effects of tuina massage techniques are not contingent solely upon the intensity of the stimulus but also upon the site of stimulus application — the acupoint. When tuina is applied to acupoints it brings about the acupuncture sensation or de Qi and the sensory stimulus generated that follows in principle the same pathway along the CNS as the acupuncture stimulus.

• C H A P T E R   V I I I •

NURTURING LIFE
养生

WHAT IS 'NURTURING LIFE' OR, IN CHINESE, 'YANG SHENG'? 'YANG' 养 LITERALLY means to nurture, while 'sheng' 生 means 'life', being a symbol of a continuously growing plant. Hence 'yang sheng' literally means 'to nurture life'.

'Nurturing life' or 'yang sheng' refers to a two-thousand-year-old body of TCM knowledge detailing concepts, practices, life experiences and lifestyles which aim at disease prevention, good health and longevity. In short, nurturing life is TCM's art of longevity and good health.

THE YIN AND YANG OF NURTURING LIFE

Chinese philosophy puts a premium on maintaining a balance between the antagonistic but inter-dependent features of a myriad of phenomena in the universe represented by the concept of yin and yang. Day (yang) is followed by night (yin); hot (yang) must be balanced by cold (yin); fire (yang) must be balanced by water (yin); and the spirit (yang) must be balanced by the physical body (yin). A relative balance or equilibrium must always be maintained between yin and yang. Disruption in this balance or disequilibrium will lead to chaos, abnormal phenomena in nature and disease.

In the archaic Chinese language, nature is termed as 'tian di' or 'heaven-earth'. Ancient philosophers saw heaven from which the yang Qi emanates as situated above, and the earth from which the yin Qi emanates as situated below. Standing between them is the human being, the product of the interaction between the yin and yang Qi from heaven and earth. The human being is a mirror image of nature itself and the laws and forces of nature, i.e. the regular pattern of yin and yang interaction, operates and pervades human beings. In order to survive, to maintain health and prevent the ravages of disease, humankind must master these laws.

THE FOUR SEASONS

The first law of nature to master is the law of the four seasons, the change from one season to another, the transformation of yin and yang. The whole year is seen as a cycle of warm spring, hot summer, cool autumn and cold winter. Warm and hot weather are considered yang, while cool and cold weather are yin. The normal alternating pattern of weather changes during the four seasons are favourable conditions for growth and development of all living things. However, weather changes are far more varied than this. Generally speaking, it is windy in spring, hot and clammy in summer, dry in autumn and cold in winter. Human beings must harmonise with the yin and yang transformations of the four seasons in order to maintain and optimise their wellbeing.

Patterns of acute and drastic weather changes, i.e. extremes in seasonal changes, can become favourable conditions for the emergence and development of diseases. For example, exposure to cold elements during winter can affect the exterior of the body and bring about a cold external clinical pattern. Hence to prevent illnesses, one must take measures to cope with extremes in seasonal changes.

Spring

Spring is the season when life begins and everything starts to develop and flourish. Flowers bloom and insects formerly in hibernation become active. Each day of this season must be treasured. Spiritually, one should harmonise with the liveliness of spring, think pleasant thoughts as if one can live without dying, as if one can give away all without losing anything, or as if one can take rewards without expecting any obligation. This will enliven and envigorate the spirit.

At the start of the day, wake up earlier, take a walk and do more outdoor activities, especially physical exercise. In the evening, sleep a little later than usual. During spring, eat more sweet and less sour-flavoured foods to nourish the spleen system which, like the soil during the spring season, needs the tonifying and nourishing attributes of sweet foods to promote growth and transformation. Avoid too much alchohol and oily, rich foods which are difficult to digest.

Summer

Summer is the season of growth when a myriad of living things flourish and become luxuriant. It is the season when the yang Qi from heaven descends and the fire from earth ascends. Spiritually, strive to stay calm and avoid anger. Rise early in the morning and sleep a little later at night. It is best to eat light, low-fat and easily digested foods. Eat more summer season fruits and melons which are mainly cooling and cold in attributes.

Summer is the hottest of all seasons. During this time, people perspire a lot, feel thirsty, expend a lot of energy and lose appetite, sleep and weight. Hence have more drinks with cooling attributes, e.g. watermelon juice, soya milk and mung bean soup.

Autumn

Autumn is the season of ripening and harvesting. The sky is high and the atmosphere tense. The yang Qi gradually eclipses while the yin Qi peaks. The weather changes from hot to cold, gradually turning cool during mornings and evenings.

During autumn, rise and sleep early. Keep the spirit tranquil, comfortable and easy as this will help cushion the clearing-away (clearing of leaves from trees) atmosphere of autumn. When autumn begins and the weather starts to cool, autumn fruits, melons and cold drinks should not be eaten in large quantities. This can bring about accumulation of phlegm and heat inside the body leading to illness. Because of the changing weather, pay attention to keeping warm. Attacks by pathogenic factors of cold must be avoided during autumn.

Winter
Winter is the season of hibernation, the coldest of the four seasons. After reaching its peak, the yin Qi starts to wane while the yang Qi starts to grow. Plants and trees wither and insects hibernate.

Sleep early at night and rise later than usual. Sunrise and sunset should be taken as the standard for the time to sleep and wake up. If one has made some gains spiritually, try to sustain that feeling. Keep the spirit tranquil. Physically, do not disturb the yang Qi of the body, avoid extreme cold and maintain body warmth.

Winter is the season to tonify and strengthen the body. People who are physically weak and convalescing from illness must take advantage of winter to tonify the body in order to have a stronger physical foundation for the coming year.

Tonifying can be achieved through foods or through medicinal herbs. There is a Chinese saying, tonifying through medicinal herbs is not as good as tonifying through the food we eat'. The most common foods taken for tonifying purposes are mutton, chicken, shark fin, sea cucumber, swallows nest, eggs and soya milk. However, the intake of this food must still suit the presenting condition of the person concerned.

UNITY OF BODY AND SPIRIT

One of the basic principles of Nurturing Life is the 'oneness and unity of the body and the spirit' or 'xing shen he yi' 形神合一 This means combining the physical and mental or combining the physical form with its functional and spiritual manifestations. The body aspect includes the various organ and channel systems as well as the body tissues, while the spirit includes all the activities of the mind and consciousness. Like the contradictory but complementary aspects of yin and yang, the body (yin) and spirit (yang) are closely and symbiotically linked. Neither can exist independently.

According to the ancient Chinese classic, *Text On the Withering of the Spirit*, 'the spirit is the body and the body is the spirit. If the body exists, then the spirit exists'. To achieve oneness and unity of the body and the spirit, the spirit must be nurtured and the body regulated. In this way, longevity can be achieved.

Nurturing the Spirit
There is a common Chinese saying which goes, 'A full and vigorous spirit is the symbol of good health'. A full and vibrant spirit promotes the normal functioning of the body's Qi, blood and organ systems and vice versa. If one is in poor spirits, negative emotions emerge and develop and a 'hundred illnesses' will result. As the *Canon On Medicine* states, 'If the spirit is preserved from within

and nurtured well, then the body's anti-pathogenic Qi [body's resistance to ill-ness] will be strong. One's flesh and skin pores will be sturdy and pathogenic factors like wind will not easily cause havoc on the body'.

Maintaining a tranquil mind is the best way to nurture the spirit, preserving its vigour and fullness. It is said that 'tranquillity leads to longevity while impetuosity leads to premature death'. To achieve tranquillity of the mind, have an even temper, always proceed from reality and avoid wild flights of fancy, do not harbour any misgivings and avoid blind optimism. Control and regulate one's obsessive desires to facilitate concentration so that the spirit is preserved. If the spirit is preserved, then the mind will be tranquil; and if the mind is tran-quil the body functions will be normal.

Keeping the emotions within normal limits is another way of nurturing the spirit. This means that emotions and feelings must not be allowed to over-react, as extreme fluctuations in emotional response to stimuli can affect the normal functioning of the major organ systems of the body.

The Seven Emotions

TCM identifies the 'seven emotions' of happiness, anger, worry, pensiveness, sadness, fear and terror as normal human spiritual expressions. However, under certain circumstances, sudden emotional fluctuations, i.e. being too angry, too sad, too terrified, and so on, which exceeds the normal sphere of control, can affect the circulation of Qi which eventually affects the normal functioning of the organ and channel systems of the body.

The Qi is the most basic substance which makes up the universe. It per-vades the cosmos and the human body, in which it circulates, interconnects and nourishes to maintain health. Excessive anger can make the Qi surge upwards; excessive worry depresses its flow; too much joy or happiness slows its circula-tion; excessive grief dispels it; excessive pensiveness causes it to coalesce into a knot and cause obstruction; fear makes it descend dramatically; while terror or fright creates chaotic Qi movement.

Extreme anger can affect the liver organ system as it can make the liver Qi rise bringing about a clinical pattern with symptoms of chest congestion, pain and congestion along both flanks, dizziness and loss of appetite.

Grief or extreme sadness can affect the normal functioning of the lung sys-tem which, in addition to its respiratory functions, is also responsible for the cir-culation of Qi all over the body. Extreme sadness can bring about disharmony in Qi circulation and a clinical pattern with symptoms of lack of energy, dis-comfort in breathing and coughing.

Extreme worry and pensiveness can harm the spleen system responsible for the transformation and transportation of food. Constant brooding and worry-ing causes 'idleness of the stomach', a clinical pattern characterised by loss of appetite.

Excessive fright can affect the normal functioning of the kidney system which in TCM is responsible for reproduction, regeneration and the excretion of body waste. Excessive fright often leads to a weakness all over the body and sometimes stool and urine incontinence. This phenomenon is known in TCM as 'fright bringing about the downward movement of the Qi'.

Terror can affect the normal functioning of the heart system which 'houses the spirit'. Terror can cause a loss of tranquillity which can lead to nervous disorders.

Happiness is the manifestation of pleasant feelings which are beneficial to the body. However, extreme happiness can be harmful to the heart system, as it can lead to uneasiness and a loss of tranquillity, appetite and sleep.

Balancing Emotional Extremes

To address clinical patterns brought about by extremes of emotions, TCM prescribes a careful balancing.

As the Qi dramatically surges upward as a result of anger, the counteracting emotional therapy of grief is used to dispel it. Excessive worry leads to a depressed and trapped Qi, hence happiness is prescribed to facilitate the Qi's smooth flow. Excessive grief and sadness which dispel Qi can be rectified by the emotion of happiness. Fear dramatically moves the Qi downwards, hence the emotion of pensiveness which knots the flow of Qi is used to restore harmony. Pensiveness and brooding over a particular problem can obstruct the free flow of Qi thereby stagnating it, so the counter-balancing emotion of anger which moves the Qi upwards and dispels Qi obstruction, is used. Finally, fright which causes the Qi to move in a chaotic direction, is balanced by the emotion of worry which traps and depresses Qi.

Regulating the Body

Nurturing the spirit can keep the body healthy which in turn promotes spiritual wellbeing as the body is the repository of the spirit. Only when the body is complete and perfect, can the spirit manifest itself. The *Canon on Medicine* states, 'If the body is not worn out then the spirit will not disperse'.

Hence in safeguarding one's wellbeing, not only nurture the spirit but give sufficient care to the body through sound diet, nutrition and a regulated life rhythm (including a moderate sex life and physical exercise).

Diet and Nutrition

The Tang-dynasty (618–907) medical scholar Sun Zi Miao said: 'The foundation of life and tranquillity comes from food. Those who do not know how to eat properly do not deserve to live'. Food and water are the source from which the vital essence of all the organ systems of the body are replenished. Food is also the raw material from which the Qi and blood is produced. Hence, food is the 'foundation of life'.

While the vital role of food is universally accepted, it can also hamper the road to health and wellbeing if not taken properly. Eating properly means regulated eating, of which there are two aspects: regulating the amount of food intake and proper food blending.

Dietary Pattern

Food must be taken in appropriate quantities, at appropriate times and must follow a definite pattern. Increasing one's food intake dramatically can injure the stomach and intestine systems. A Ming-dynasty (1368–1644) medical scholar lists the 'five illnesses' resulting from overeating: frequent bowel movements, frequent urination, too much sleep, lack of concentration and frequent indigestion.

The Chinese say that it is best to 'Eat well at breakfast, eat to the full at lunch and eat less at dinner'. This is similar to the English saying, 'Eat like a king at breakfast; eat like a queen at lunchtime; and eat like a pauper at dinnertime'.

In the morning, if one's appetite is poor, choose food which is small in volume but full of calories to keep one going for the day's work. At lunchtime, eat to the full. Choose food rich in protein with some small amount of oil and fat to supplement energy expended in the morning and to prepare for the afternoon's work.

Calorie consumption at night should be low. Take easily digested food such as vegetables and some food containing natural sugars. From ancient times, eating less during dinner time has been a constant Chinese practice. There is a Chinese saying which goes, 'A mouthful of food less at dinner time can make one live to ninety-nine'.

In the evening, when asleep, the level of activity is very low. If there is too much intake of nutritious food, there will be an over-supply of calories which in turn will be stored as fat. In addition, over-eating at dinner can increase the burden on the stomach and intestines, resulting in a feeling of abdominal distention and possible indigestion which can in turn, influence sleep.

In general, it is best to form the habit of eating three meals a day, five to six hours apart, with nothing taken in between. Generally speaking, mixed foods stay within the stomach for four to five hours. For the remaining time, the digestive organs need to rest in order to regain their normal function.

Food Blending — You Are What You Eat!

In the chapter on Food Therapy, the various attributes of foods, i.e. flavours and Qi attributes, are discussed. These attributes have to be considered in the choice of food. In addition, food flavours also favour certain system inclinations. For example, sour-flavoured foods are inclined to favour the liver system; bitter-flavoured foods favour the heart organ system; sweet foods favour the spleen system; pungent-flavoured foods favour the lung system; and the salty ones favour the kidney organ system. In order to achieve total body nourishment, foods of various flavours and Qi attributes must be combined and blended to suit the individual's body constitution, clinical pattern and lifestyle.

People who have a hot body constitution or clinical pattern must eat foods which are generally cool or cold in Qi attribute. If they have a kidney deficiency they should eat more salty-flavoured food. Those with a cold body constitution or clinical pattern, should eat foods with warm or hot attributes, while those with lung system problems must eat more pungent-flavoured foods. This principle guides one to select and combine food in accordance with one's respective physical condition.

It also prevents partiality to one particular food, i.e. eating or drinking too much of a particular food, such as alcohol, coffee, chocolate or fried or junk food, without regard to the consequences. Because each food type has its respective flavour, Qi attribute and organ system inclination, having one type of food for a protracted time can lead to illness. For example, too much food with a pungent flavour and a hot Qi attribute, like scallions and ginger, or too much oily food with a sweet flavour, will lead to the build up of heat and dampness in the body and manifest itself as a hot clinical pattern. Coffee (a warm and sweet flavour with a therapeutic attribute of 'stimulating the spirit'), when taken excessively, can build up heat in the body and affect sleep.

To bring about a healthy balance and harmony among the various organ systems of the body, TCM dietary principles also advocate eating mixed foods with a high proportion of grain as energy-giving foods. Protein intake should come mainly from beans and legumes and their by-products. Only very little animal and oily food should be taken.

A survey completed in China on people aged more than a hundred revealed that most ate mixed grains (rice, millet, wheat and beans) with a variety of vegetables as their main staple food. None were overweight.

TCM dietary principles also stress a moderate intake of light food rather than oily and highly concentrated food. 'Rich and nutritious food and the drinking of strong liquor are the main causes of disease', states the ancient classic *Lu Shi In Spring and Autumn*.

The accumulation of dampness, mucus and phlegm within the body are attributed to the over-eating of meat, oily, fried and hot food, as well as to too much alcohol. This condition eventually leads to what is termed as 'liver-wind clinical pattern', the symptoms and signs of which are found among patients who suffer from hypertension, coronary heart disease and stroke.

Regulated Life Rhythm

Nature has its own rhythms and patterns of motion, as does the human body. A regular pattern and rhythm promote good health, whereas the opposite leads to disharmony and hence disease among the organ systems of the body. Insomnia, for example, can result from prolonged shift work which upsets the natural rhythm of work, rest and sleep.

The TCM concept of nurturing life stresses the importance of adjusting to or harmonising with the natural environment, i.e. night and day; the pace of life;

seasonal and weather changes; economic, political and societal changes, etc. A rhythm in daily life with appropriate alternation of work, rest, recreation, eating, sleep, exercise, social interaction etc, harmonised with nature, is essential.

Sleep

One important element for a regular rhythm is sleep. A 'natural tonic', it can eliminate fatigue, make up for wear and tear and restore nutritional absorption. The time given to sleep means energy gained for tomorrow's work. In the course of a person's life, about one third of the time is spent sleeping.

To achieve depth and a reasonable duration of sleep, establish a regular sleeping habit. Definite sleeping and waking times are very important, as is a tranquil and relaxed mind before sleep. The ancient Chinese book *Sleeping Techniques* written during the Song Dynasty (960–1279) states: 'Sleep with curled body on one side. Straighten ... when waking up. Sleep at definite times at night and wake up at definite times in the morning. First make the mind sleep and then make the eyes sleep'.

The body's position during sleep has some bearing on the quality of the sleep. During ancient times, it was believed that sleeping on the right side 'curled like a bow' was best. One popular method for aiding sleep is to wash both feet in a basin of warm to hot water. This method is thought to bring the blood from the head down to the feet and thus facilitate sleep. Most nurturing life experts agree that the bed head should face the eastern direction during spring and summer and face the west during autumn and winter.

Spring and summer, and the eastern aspect has a preponderance of yang Qi which corresponds to an ascending direction. By placing the head in the eastern direction during these seasons, one can harmonise with the nourishing and ascending yang Qi. Thus this will be beneficial for sleep. Conversely, during autumn and winter a western aspect has a preponderance of yin Qi with a descending direction, so if the head faces west, it harmonises with a nourishing yin Qi.

Regulated Sex Life

According to TCM, the kidney system is mainly responsible for reproductive functions. This system stores the 'constitutional essence' or jing which acts as the structural foundation and sustains the kidney and the rest of the body's organ systems. The constitutional essence, inherited from the parents and from food nutrients, sustains the reproductive and sexual activities, produces semen and sustains the menstrual cycle.

In this context, preserving the 'constitutional essence' of the kidney system through regulated sexual and reproductive activities promotes longevity. Conversely, protracted over-indulgence in sexual activities can exhaust the 'constitutional essence' and lead to a clinical pattern known as kidney system deficiency. The main signs and symptoms of this clinical pattern are: lower back pains, dizziness, tinnitus, lack of spirit, wet dreams, impotency, irregular periods, and excessive vaginal discharge. Emaciation and premature ageing can also result from an over-active sex life.

Among the medical classics written on bamboo strips unearthed in China in 1973 from the Ma Wang Dui Tomb in Changsha, was a chapter called 'Discussions On The Tao Of the Land' (circa 168 BC). This chapter included specific instructions on beneficial sexual practices to maintain a healthy kidney system.

First: Regulate the Qi before sexual intercourse. Do Qi Gong exercises (discussed later in the chapter) to free up the flow of Qi and blood throughout the body.

Second: Frothing the body fluids. The frequent swallowing of saliva accumulated under the tongue can strengthen the body. Increased vaginal and penile secretions facilitate the conduct of sexual intercourse.

Third: Timing. Be good at grasping the right time for intercourse.

Fourth: Storing the Qi. To store the 'constitutional essence' and Qi, the male must hold back ejaculation.

Fifth: Union of the froth. Perfect coordination during sexual intercourse between the male and the female occurs with the swallowing of saliva from under the tongue and the generation of body fluids.

Sixth: Accumulating Qi. An appropriate end to sexual intercourse will prevent fatigue and thus accumulate more constitutional essence and Qi.

Seventh: Maintain a brimming constitutional essence and Qi. During intercourse leave some room to manoeuvre, maintain a full constitutional essence and Qi so as not to lead to kidney system deficiency.

Eighth: Prevent ecstasy. During intercourse the man should not be ecstatic but maintain control.

Seven harmful sexual practices are listed. These are:

First: Internal obstruction. Do not have sex if there is penile pain or obstruction of the semen duct, which may lead to failure to ejaculate.

Second: External emission of the yang Qi, i.e. uncontrolled sweating during intercourse.

Third: Exhaustion. Unregulated sex life with unlimited sexual intercourse can lead to the exhaustion of the constitutional essence.

Fourth: Loss of erection during intercourse.

Fifth: Trouble during intercourse, the feeling of breathlessness, panting, upset or confusion.

Sixth: Reaching an impasse. This occurs when the female has no sexual urge and the male becomes impetuous and forces intercourse. Such action will damage the woman's spirit and body and affect the future foetus.

Seventh: Haste. During intercourse a quick and hurried ejaculation is wasteful, and leads to the exhaustion of constitutional essence and the Qi.

According to the chapter on 'Discussions on the Tao of the Land', in order to increase one's longevity and postpone ageing, one must use the 'Eight Beneficial Sexual Practices' to strengthen the body. In this way old people recover their youth, while the young will not easily age.

Physical Exercise

One of the most important methods of nurturing the body is through physical movement. 'Motion prevents (physical) decline', as one Chinese saying goes. The ancient literary classic, *Lu Shi's Spring and Autumn Annals* states, 'Running water is never stagnant and a door hinge never gets worm-eaten. This is what motion is all about ... If the body does not move then the constitutional essence (jing) will not flow. And if the constitutional essence does not flow then Qi flow stagnates'.

The *Canon On Medicine* extended this concept to the workings of the human body by stating that if any part of the body is not moved then the Qi will not circulate, leading to stagnation. If this occurs in the head, there will be swelling; if in the ears, there will be hearing loss; if in the eyes, eyesight deteriorates; and if in the nose, it becomes blocked; if in the abdomen, it becomes distended; and if in the extremities, atrophy results. Physical exercise therefore is an integral part of TCM concepts and practices for nurturing life. Its purpose is to strengthen the body, prevent disease and achieve longevity.

Physical exercise can hamonise the body (yin) and the spirit (yang) as well as the Qi (yang) and the constitutional essence (yin). These in turn are beneficial to the internal harmony between the various organ systems, as well as between the body and the natural environment.

Chinese traditional physical exercises have three main characteristics and requirements. First, there must be a harmonious unity between mental imaging or yi shou 意守, regulated breathing or tiao xi 调息 and body postures and movements or dong xing 动形. Second, they must be performed appropriately and not to excess. Third, perseverance in practising them is essential.

Mental Imaging *Yi Shou* 意守

The Chinese term for mental imaging 'yi shou' literally means to hold on to an image or idea. It refers to focusing one's mind upon an image, idea or thought which may be an acupoint, a special area of the body like the 'elixir field' or 'dan tian' (a spot under the umbilicus) or the flow of Qi along an acupuncture channel. The idea to be focused upon may be outside the body, e.g. a beautiful natural landscape or a flower. Successful mental imaging comes from long practice. It also comes from a tranquil spirit which is free from any distractions or obsessions. A focused mind promotes nurturing of the spirit.

Regulated Breathing *Tiao Xi* 调息

Regulated breathing refers to controlled inhalation and exhalation of the Qi which comes from the air we breathe. When this Qi combines in the chest with the Qi transformed from the food and water we digest, another type of Qi, 'essential Qi, is formed. The essential Qi flows into the heart and lung channels and into the pharynx and larynx before moving down into the 'elixir field'.

The essential Qi regulates respiration and promotes blood circulation. To regulate breathing, various techniques are employed. These are the natural breathing method, abdominal breathing, deep breathing, mouth exhalation and nasal inhalation breathing technique, nasal inhalation and exhalation technique and intermittent breathing techniques.

Body Movements *Dong Xing* 动形

Every posture or body movement influences and promotes the flow of Qi and blood along the channels and internal organ systems. Every movement therefore does not only have a localised effect. For example, movement of the four extremities is beneficial to the spleen system and digestion. Movement of the lower back is good for the kidney system and reproductive functions. Movement of the eyes is good not only for these organs but also for the liver system.

Body movements may be slow as in Tai Chi or Qi Gong or they can be quick and strong as in the martial arts movements. The first step in any TCM exercise is to adjust the posture. This regulates the breathing and mental imaging. Mental imaging, body movements and breathing must be done harmoniously in a unified manner. The mental imaging nurtures the spirit, breathing tempers the Qi, while body movements faciliate Qi and blood circulation in the various channels. Mental imaging guides the Qi, while the Qi moves throughout the body.

When exercising, the spirit and internal organ systems are nurtured, while externally the channels, bones, sinews, four extremities and tendons are exercised. This results in the unity and harmony between the internal and external regions of the body, the smooth circulation of the Qi and blood, and a unified spirit and body all of which results in a harmonious interaction between the yin and yang aspects of the body. The important requirement for physical exercise is finding the optimum amount one needs. If it is too little, then it is ineffective, if it is too much then fatigue or injury can result. So, to determine the optimum level, physical exercise must be done in a gradual manner.

Perseverance is another important factor for physical exercise. Once started, it must be done continuously. 'A continuously flowing water never stagnates', the saying goes. 'Fishing for three days while drying the net for two days' will not achieve the purpose of physical exercise. Exercise not only tempers the body, but more importantly the will and determination.

Various Types of Traditional Physical Exercises
There are various types of traditional physical exercise for nurturing life. All have the three elements explained earlier but differ in some theoretical under-pinings or movements. Traditional physical exercises most commonly known in the West are Qi Gong and Tai Chi.

Qi Gong 气功 can literally be translated as 'skill in harnessing the Qi'. It is an exercise which puts more stress on mental imaging and breathing and less on movement. Common body postures used are sitting and standing.

Qi Gong may be categorised into a Taoist or Confucian type, depending upon its philosophical basis. Qi Gong can also be combined with martial arts. There are many varieties of Qi Gong exercises, such as relaxation Qi Gong, internal nurturing Qi Gong, body strengthening Qi Gong, tranquillity Qi Gong.

Qi Gong can also be used in healing. This may be done in two ways. A patient can learn a specific Qi Gong exercise to address his or her clinical pattern or a TCM practitioner harnesses his or her own Qi and uses this to har-monise the flow of Qi in patients.

Taijiquan 太极拳 is more often referred to in the West as 'Tai Chi'. The term 'taiji' refers to the borderline separating the black (yin) and white (yang) in the yin and yang symbol. It is the climactic phase or stage when yin or yang transforms into its opposite. 'Quan' refers to the movement of the fist as in shadow boxing.

Tai Chi is a physical exercise involving the continuous movement of the four extremities, the head, spine and eyes, combined with breathing and men-tal imaging. Compared to Qi Gong, it places more emphasis on movement.

Tai Chi can ease joint movement and harmonise the flow of the Qi. In exer-cising the body, it has the effect of strengthening it and preventing diseases. There are many Tai Chi styles, e.g. Yang, Chen and Wu styles.

The five animals exercises *Wu Qin Xi* 五禽戏
The Five Animals Exercises are one of the oldest sets of continuously practised traditional physical exercises in China. They combine the elements of breath-ing, image focusing and physical movements. The physical movement mimics those of the tiger, bear, monkey, deer and the crane, hence the name. The men-tal imaging is primarily focused upon important acupoints.

When this set of physical exercises is performed regularly, the general ben-efits are to nourish the spirit, regulate Qi and blood flow, promote circulation along the channels and enliven the movement of the tendons, joints and bones.

The Five Animals Exercises were developed during the later Han Dynasty by an ancient medical scholar called Hua Tuo. According to historical records a disciple who persisted in doing this exercise lived for more than 90 years, while still retaining good hearing, eyesight and a complete set of teeth.

There are four key movements for all animal forms

1. Relaxation: First of all, relax the entire body, feel light and optimistic so as to facilitate the smooth flow of Qi and blood, and reinvigorate the spirit. Relaxation also prevents tension and any stiffness in movement.

2. Even breathing: Breathing must be calm and natural. Use abdominal breathing which should be done evenly, calmly and slowly. When breathing, the mouth must be almost closed with the tip of the tongue touching the upper palate. Inhale through the nose and exhale through the mouth.

3. Mental imaging: All mental distractions must be discarded. Focus on the required mental image to achieve coordination between the Qi and the mind.

4. Natural movement: Each animal requires a specific type of movement. For example, the bear is heavy and slow; the monkey is light and nimble; the tiger is strong and firm; the deer is tame and meek; while the bird is very active. Execute the movements naturally in accordance with the characteristics of each animal.

The Tiger Form

1. Mimicking the tiger: Mimic the tiger's strong clawing power and express its powerful and fierce bearing, flashing eyes, shaking head and swaying tail, as if mounting a lunging attack.

2. Mental imaging: Focus mentally on the acupoint Gate of Life (a point in between the 2nd and 3rd lumbar vertebrae) to strengthen the kidney organ system and the lower back.

3. Preparatory movements: Stand erect naturally and relax. Heels must be placed together. Keep mouth slightly open, while the tongue tip touches the upper palate. Breath naturally and evenly.

4. Movement to the left side: Bend both knees in half squatting position. Weight must be on right leg. Raise the left leg slightly and then place it beside the right ankle joint with the ball of the foot lightly touching the ground. Clench both fists, facing upwards, and raise them to the sides of the waist. Look forward towards the left at a 45 degree angle.

5. Slowly and gradually inhale the Qi. With both fists facing the body, raise them above the chest to the front of the mouth. Exhale the Qi. Turn the fists

outwards and open them as you move the hands forward in a pressing down direction. At the same time, move the left foot towards the left forward direction. The ball of the left foot touches the ground becoming a slight step, while the right foot follows half a step in the same direction. Both heels must be level, with a distance of one foot separating them. Your weight must be centered upon your right foot. The eyes must look at the tip of the left index finger.

6. Movement to the right side: Move the left foot slightly forward in a half step. The right foot follows touching the ankle joint of the left foot. Raise the right foot slightly so that its ball is still touching the ground. Clench both fists and raise them to waist level, then face the fists upwards. The eyes must look forwards towards the right.

7. Slowly inhale the Qi. Raise your clenched fists to your chest with the fists facing upwards. When the fists reach the front of the mouth, exhale the Qi. Turn the fists outward and open while moving them in a forward pushing down manner. At the same time, move the right foot forward one step towards the right. The left foot follows half a step in the same direction. Place both heels side by side a foot apart. Weight must fall upon the left foot. The right foot slightly touches the ground and become a slight step. The eyes must look at the tip of the right index finger.

Note: When doing this exercise, the breathing and movements must be coordinated. When both hands are turned outwards and pressed in a downward direction, both legs must move forward at the same time. At this point a slight force can be used. The speed must be quick to mimic the agility of a lunging tiger.

The Deer Form

1. Mimicking the deer: The nimble and long-living deer is good at swaying its tail and rear. Moving these regions of the body can promote the inter-connection of the two acupuncture channels which run along the middle section of the abdomen and back. In executing the Deer Form, you are mimicking its spiritual tranquillity, as well as its smooth and lithe body form. The deer's characteristics of stretching out, its run, upright neck, and the way it turns its head must be manifested in the exercise.

2. Mental imaging: Focus mentally upon the sacral and coccyx area, to promote the circulation of Qi and blood throughout the body and to stretch the tendons and bones.

3. Preparatory movements: Both feet are slightly apart level with both shoulders, both arms at the sides. Relax, breathe evenly and calmly.

4. Bend the right knee while moving the upper torso backwards. Stretch the left leg forward while the knee is slightly bent, with the left foot lightly touching the ground. Stretch both hands with both elbows slightly bent, the left hand in front while placing the right hand on the inner side of the left elbow. Both palms face each other.

5. Rotate the waist, hip and the sacral region in an anti-clockwise direction with arms and hands following. The hands and arms make a big rotational movement, while the sacral joints execute a small rotational movement. This is is the 'deer rotating the sacral area' movement.

6. Shift your weight to the left leg. With the right leg, make a step forward and stretch the right hand forward, while placing the left hand over on the inner side of the right elbow. In a clockwise direction rotate the waist, hip and sacral joint taking with it both hands and arms to execute a rotational movement in front of the body. Repeat in the the other direction.

Note: The rotation of the hand and forearm relies upon the rotational movement of the waist, hip and sacral region. This is not a shoulder joint movement. This movement can benefit the kidney system and strengthen the lower back, as well as enliven blood circulation in the pelvic region. It can also relax the tendons and bones.

The Bear Form

1. Mimicking the bear: Mimic the bear's huge body and powerful strength which is tranquil on the outside but seething with activity within. Embody the bear's simplicity, vigour, heaviness and steadiness. Express its earth-shaking and ambulatory way of walking which, although appearing heavy and cumbersome, is also full of nimbleness.
   The Bear Form is beneficial for upper deficiency and lower excess clinical patterns. It can overcome the feeling of heaviness in the head and lightness in the extremities, and strengthen the various internal organ systems.

2. Mental imaging: When doing this exercise focus on the inner umbilicus while making the Qi sink into the elixir field.

3. Preparatory movements: Stand naturally erect with both feet apart and level with both shoulders. Dangle both arms at the side. Breathe evenly and calmly. Mentally focus upon the inner umbilicus to regulate Qi and blood flow. Focus on external tranquillity but internal activity, make the spirit tranquil, merge the Qi and mind.

4. Exhale the Qi while slowly moving the left foot half a step forward towards the left. With the waist as the axis of the movement, rotate the waist slightly

towards the left side of the body. Move the left shoulder towards the outer back direction while the arm is bent. At the same time, bend the right knee and, following the rotational movement of the upper torso, rock the right shoulder in a forward and downward direction, with the arm dangling by the side of the body following this movement. At this point, weight should be on the right leg.

5. As one inhales the Qi, rotate the body slightly towards the right direction. Gradually shift your weight from the right leg to the left leg. Keep the right foot on the inner side of the left foot.

6. Exhale while slowly moving the right leg half a step forward towards the right. With the waist as the axis, rotate the trunk to the right, while spreading the right shoulder towards the outer and back. Slightly bend the elbow. At the same time, bend the left knee, rock the right shoulder towards the front lower direction and move the hand and arm to the side of the body.

7. Inhale while rotating the body slightly towards the right side. Gradually shift your weight from the left leg to the right leg. Move the left foot to the inner side of the right foot.

Note: The movement must be steady, heavy and slow. In mimicking the vigorous movements of the bear, alternate between the left and right and rock the body repeatedly.

Monkey Form

1. Mimic the monkey: Mimic the monkey's alertness, agility nimbleness and activity. Express its character as seen when it jumps up and down a mountain, climbs trees and branches, picks fruits and offers them. The Monkey Form develops flexibility.

2. Mental imaging: Focus on the mental image of the inner umbilicus to attain physical activity and tranquillity of the spirit. When focusing, exercise the flexibility of the extremities on the outside and the tranquillity of the spirit internally.

3. Preparatory movements: Stand erect naturally and relax. Slightly close the mouth while placing the tip of the tongue on the upper palate. Breath evenly.

4. Slowly bend both knees and shift the weight of the body to the right leg. Move the left leg lightly and nimbly towards the front, while simultaneously moving the left hand level with the mouth via the front of the chest. Stretch the hand forward as if to take something. When the hand reaches the front

of the mouth, change the hand into a grasping form as you naturally drop the wrist. The centre of the body weight must be shifted to the left foot.

5. Move the right foot slowly and lightly towards the front. Gradually move weight onto the right foot. Raise the left heel so the sole touches the ground very lightly. Simultaneously raise the right hand to mouth level, passing the front of the chest. Stretch the hand forward as if to take something. When the hand reaches mouth level, assume a grasping form while dropping the wrist naturally. Simultaneously move the left hand back to the left side of the waist.

6. Make the body sit towards the back. Gradually shift weight from the right to the left foot. Slightly move the left foot backwards, make it steady, then move the right foot backwards, with the ball of the foot touching the ground. At the same time, raise the left hand and pass it along the front of the chest. Stretch it forward like taking something. When the hand reaches mouth level, change the palm into a grasping hold and naturally drop the wrist. At the same time move the right hand to the side of the waist.

7. Move the right leg lightly and nimbly towards the front, while simultaneously moving the right hand level with the mouth via the front of the chest. Stretch the hand forward as if taking something. When the hand reaches the front of the mouth, change the hand into a grasping form as you naturally drop the wrist.

8. Move the left foot slowly and lightly towards the front. Following this movement, raise the right foot so that the ball touches the ground very lightly. Simultaneously, raise the right hand level with the mouth passing through the front of the chest. Stretch the hand forward as if to take something. When the hand reaches the mouth level, assume a grasping form while dropping the wrist naturally. Bring the right hand towards the flank.

9. Make the body sit towards the back. Slightly move the right foot backwards, make it steady, then move the left foot backwards with the ball of the foot touching the ground. At the same time raise the right hand passing along the front of the chest. Stretch it forward like taking something. When it reaches the mouth level, change the palm into a grasping hold and naturally drop the wrist. Bring the left hand back to the flank.

Note: When inhaling, only partially open the lips, to just allow the air to pass through the teeth. When exhaling use the mouth to gradually expel the Qi.

Crane Form

1. Mimicking the crane: Mimic the crane's light movement, its limbering up,

spreading of feathers and flight. Be upright, tall, straight, carefree and contented. Express its bearing of having bright feathers, easy flight and independence.

2. Mental imaging: Focus mentally the 'Sea of Qi' acupoint located about one and half inches below the navel, the point from where all the Qi emanates. This exercise can promote Qi and blood flow as well as move the joints and bones. The crane exercise can also strengthen the lung respiratory function.

3. Preparatory movements: Place both feet side by side and stand naturally erect. Fix the vision forward and relax.

4. Move the left foot forward one step, move the right foot to follow about half a step, touch the ground very lightly. Place weight on the left foot. Simultaneously raise both arms along the sides of the body. When raising the arms inhale deeply.

5. Move the right foot forward half a step, place next to the left foot. Drop both arms from left and right sides. While exhaling very deeply, bend both knees, and use arms to hold both knees.

6. Move the right foot one step forward, move the left foot to follow half a step forward with the left foot touching the ground very lightly. Place weight on the right foot. Raise both arms along left and right sides while inhaling deeply.

7. Move the left foot forward half a step and place it side by side with right foot. Drop both left and right arms along the sides of the body. Bend the knees while at the same time exhaling deeply. Use the arms to embrace both knees.

The movements must be coordinated with breathing. Inhale when stretching out and exhale when contracting the body. The exercise may be done several times. This form can strengthen the heart and lung systems and the lower back and kidney system.

GLOSSARY OF TERMS

ACUPUNCUTURE CHANNEL NETWORK Jing Luo 经络 A network of pathways which intersects and covers all areas of the body and connects its inner and outer aspects. They are conduits through which Qi, blood and body fluids circulate through the body. There are seven of these networks.

ACCUMULATED MASS Ji Ju 积聚 A physical mass that may be palpated in the abdominal area with symptoms of pain and distention. It is triggered by emotional or dietary factors which lead to liver and spleen disharmonies. This eventually leads to blockage in Qi and blood circulation. A prolonged condition like this leads to Qi stagnation and blood stasis and thus accumulated mass.

ANTI-PATHOGENIC QI Zheng Qi 正气 'Zheng' means upright or normally functioning body, while 'Qi' is the overall manifestation of a normally functioning body, so zheng or anti-pathogenic Qi refers to the body's capacity to resist disease. Anti-pathogenic Qi also refers to the normal seasonal manifestations of winter cold or summer heat.

BIAN QUE 扁鹊 An ancient physician (500 BC) who was skilled in diagnosis, pulse-taking and acupuncture.

BLOOD Xue 血 A substance which comes from food essence and undergoes Qi transformation. This transformation occurs in the spleen and stomach systems (the middle energiser). It circulates through the blood vessels to nourish the whole body.

BLOOD DEFICIENCY CLINICAL PATTERN Xue Xu 血虚 This clinical pattern is due to deficiency in the blood production. Signs and symptons are: pale face and lips, dizziness, palpitations, inability to sleep or easily woken up, numbness in the extremities, pulse is thready and no strength.

BLOOD STASIS Xue Yu 血瘀 This is a disease pattern characterised by stagnation of blood circulation or blood flowing out of the channel orbit. It is caused by Qi stagnation, Qi deficiency, hot or cold blood, injury or trauma.

BODY FLUIDS (*See* VITAL FLUIDS)

CANON A classical text.

CHANNEL CLINICAL PATTERNS Jing Luo Bian Zheng 经络辨证 These are clinical patterns that emerge from disharmonies in the acupuncture channel system.

CLINICAL PATTERN Zheng Hou 证候 Various signs and symptoms, including pulse and tongue configuration, which emerge when a patient is sick. They are the diagnostic basis upon which therapeutic principles, methods, formulae and remedies are tailored.

CONSTITUTIONAL ESSENCE Jing 精 This is the basic substance that is derived from our parents and is nourished by food and water essence. It sustains and maintains life activities.

CUPPING Therapeutic method using glass or bamboo jars that cause local congestion. Heat is used to create a vacuum inside the jar which then placed over acupunture points. This sucks in the tissues underneath forming localised stasis.

DAMP CLINICAL PATTERN Shi Yin Zheng 湿淫证 A clinical pattern brought about by excesses in seasonal dampness affecting the body. The signs and symptoms are a feeling of heaviness all over the body, soreness in the extremities, poor appetite, diarrhoea, abdominal distention which in severe cases manifests itself as sudden swelling or fluid retention in the face and limbs.

DAMP AND PHLEGM BLOCKING CHANNEL CLINICAL PATTERN Shi Tan Zu Jing Luo Zheng 湿痰阻经络证 A spleen disharmony leading to stagnation of body fluid distribution and the resulting accumulation of phlegm. The signs and symptoms are expectoration of large quantities of whitish or yellow phlegm which may be coughed out easily, a feeling of heaviness all over the body, fatigue, abdominal distention, indigestion, abdominal pain, diarrhoea, a slippery and slow pulse. When this condition affects a particular acupuncture channel, corresponding signs and symptoms occur.

DECOCTION A herbal brew.

DEFICIENT YANG CLINICAL PATTERN Yang Xu 阳虚 A clinical pattern resulting from deficiency of the yang Qi which give rise to an internal cold clinical pattern, the signs and symptoms of which are tiredness, shortness of breath, laziness to talk, aversion to cold temperature, cold extremities, spontaneous sweating, pale face, diarrhoea, clear and prolonged urination, pale tongue, a deep, thready and big pulse.

DETOXIFYING EFFECT Jie Du Zuo Yong 解毒作用 To rid the body of toxic elements (due to pathogenic heat or cold invasion, administration of toxic substances or being exposed to them or from insect or animal bites) which have affected the blood. This can be achieved through the use of herbs or stimulating points with a detoxifying therapeutic action.

ELIXIR A herbal preparation to prolong life.

ELIXIR FIELD A spot under the umbilicus.

ENERGISER (*See* TRIPLE ENERGISER)

EXTERNAL DISEASE PATTERNS (*See* external pathogenic Qi).

EXTERNAL PATHOGENIC QI (or FACTORS) Wai Gan 外感 These are excesses in the seasonal factors of wind, heat, damp, cold, summer heat, dryness; and warm febrile diseases which can affect the body and lead to diseases.

EXTERNAL COLD-DAMP PATTERN Han Shi 寒湿 A disease brought about by the external pathogenic factors of cold and dampness, the signs and symptoms of which are pain along the muscular and superficial shell of the body and in the joints.

EXTERNAL WIND-COLD PATTERNS Feng Han Gan Mao 风寒感冒 A type of external clinical pattern which emerges when the external pathogenic factors of wind and cold affect the body, the signs and symptoms of which are body chills, a stuffy nose with watery discharge, sneezing, coughing, bone and joint aches, no thirst, whitish tongue coat, a superficial and tight pulse.

EXTERNAL WIND-HEAT PATTERN Feng Re Gan Mao 风热感冒 An external clinical pattern which emerges when the external pathogenic factors of wind and heat attack the body, the signs and symptoms of which are fever, headache, a stuffy nose without discharge, aversion to wind, spontaneous sweating, sore throat, coughing, yellow thick phlegm discharge, reddish tongue with yellow coat, a superficial and rapid pulse.

EXTREMITIES Arms and legs.

FEBRILE Feverish.

FOOD AND WATER ESSENCE Shui Gu Zhi Jing 水谷之精 The essential substance transformed from food and water, which plays a vital role in the constitution of the body and the maintenance of health and life activities. It is stored in the kidney system.

FOOD RETENTION or FOOD STAGNATION Shu Shi 宿食 or Shi Zhi 食滞 This is a clinical condition similar to symptoms of indigestion resulting from improper eating habits.

GATE OF LIFE ming men 命门 This is the right-side kidney which has been defined by the ancient classical texts as the site from which the congenital Qi or prenatal Qi (xian tian zhi Qi) originates. It is the source of life transformations, as well as the foundations of life. The 'Gate of Life' is also the name of an acupuncture point along the Governor Channel located between the 2nd and 3rd lumbar vertebral spaces.

HEAT PATHOGENIC QI (or FACTOR) Re Xie 热邪 A disease-causing factor producing signs and symptoms of fever, hoarse breathing, redness and swelling, pain accompanied by hot sensations and constipation.

HEART HOUSES THE SPIRIT Xin Zhu Shen Ming 心主神明 This refers to one of the designated functions of the heart system. The spirit here refers to one's decorum, consciousness, emotions, thinking, etc. If the heart system is functioning normally then one has a vibrant spirit and clear thinking. If not, disease clinical patterns such as forgetfulness, anxiety, sleeping problems, fear and palpitations occur.

HYPERACTIVE FIRE Huo Xing Yan Shang 火性炎上 The use of 'fire' here refers to it in the context of the Five Elements, i.e. fire flares up and razes things in the same way as a pathogenic Qi-like fire may be generated externally (from summer heat or dryness) or internally (from disharmony among the various internal organ systems like the heart or liver systems).

IDEOGRAPHIC Use of written signs or symbols for communication.

INTERNAL DISEASE QI (or FACTORS) Nei Shang 内伤 Disease-causing factors, such as excesses in emotional response, improper diet and an irregular life rhythm, all of which affect the normal functioning of the internal organ systems.

LIVER YANG HYPERACTIVITY Gan Yang Shang Kang 肝阳上亢 This is a clinical pattern characterised by dizziness, headaches, flushed face, bitter taste in the mouth, a reddish tongue and wiry pulse. It is due to the disequilibrium between the yin and yang aspects of the liver system.

MATERIA MEDICA Science of the properties of substances, their combination and use in medicine.

MIDDLE ENERGISER 'Zhong Jiao' 中焦 The middle segment of the Triple Energiser system. The middle segment includes the spleen and stomach systems.

MUCUS Shi Zhuo Zhi Xie 湿浊之邪 A pathogenic Qi with a sticky and heavy type of dampness. When it affects a particular organ system, clinical patterns with symptoms of thick and heavy mucus discharge arise.

ORBIT FLOW Movement along a pathway.

OBSTRUCTION OF THE QI Qi Zhi 气滞 This is a clinical pattern brought about by the malfunctioning of Qi circulation, characterised by localised pain or swelling and distention of one area of the body.

OPENS THE STOMACH Kai Wei 开胃 A therapeutic method which aims at improving a poor appetite with remedies like herbs or acupuncture which can promote Qi flow and boost digestion.

ORGAN SYSTEMS Wu Zang Liu Fu 五脏六腑 A re-ordering of all normal body parts and activities into five visceral and six hollow organ systems which are elucidated in the *Canons of Medicine*. The five visceral organ systems are the Heart, Liver, Spleen, Lungs and Kidneys; while the Six Hollow Organ systems are the Large Intestine, Small Intestine, Stomach, Gall Bladder, Urinary Bladder and Triple Energiser. This re-ordering of normal body parts was not based solely upon the physical and anatomical features of some of these organs. Rather, philosophical concepts were used to align the workings of these physical organs with manifestations of normal body functions and the wider external natural world.

ORIGINAL QI, SOURCE QI or PRIMORDIAL QI Yuan Qi 元气 This is one type of Qi which circulates around the body. It is the source of all life and body activities. It is transformed from the constitutional essence and is continuously nourished by food nutrients.

PATHOGENIC COLD FACTORS Han Xie 寒邪 An external pathogenic factor which possesses a yin attribute that can easily damage the yang Qi and thus influence the circulation of Qi and blood. The resulting clinical pattern has signs and symptoms of chills, fever, headache, general body ache and diarrhoea.

PATHOGENIC DAMPNESS This is similar to **DAMP CLINICAL PATTERN**

PATHOGENIC HEAT ATTACKING QI LAYER OF THE BODY Re Shang Qi 热伤气 This refers to a clinical pattern of profuse sweating brought about by the external pathogenic factor of heat invasion and affecting the Qi layer of the body responsible for opening and closing the pores of the skin.

PATHOGENIC QI Xie Qi 邪气 A generic term which refers to all disease-causing factors both external (i.e. excesses in seasonal changes) and internal (i.e. emotions, dietary factors etc). Pathogenic Qi has a symbiotic and dialectical relationship with the anti-pathogenic Qi.

PHLEGM Tan 痰 In TCM, phlegm is a product of malfunctioning lung and spleen systems and is also an internal pathogenic Qi or a factor which can cause diseases like asthma, coughing, convulsions and joint pains.

PICTOGRAPHIC Use of pictures, signs or symbols to represent an idea or concept

PYRETIC Feverish characteristics.

QI DEFICIENCY 气虚 A clinical pattern characterised by a pale facial complexion, dizziness, spontaneous sweating, shortness of breath, a weak pulse due to exhaustion of Original Qi.

QI STAGNATION *See* **OBSTRUCTION OF THE QI**

RADIAL PULSE A wrist pulse.

SIX HOLLOW ORGANS *See* **ORGAN SYSTEMS**

TONIFICATION Therapeutic methods, device, substances which can nourish that which is deficient.

TRIPLE ENERGISER San Jiao 三焦 One of the hollow organ systems which is segmented into the upper, middle and lower energiser. Each segment or region is related to a set of organ systems, hence it has the role of regulating their functions as well as regulating body fluid circulation. The upper energiser is related to the lungs and heart; the middle to the spleen and liver; and the lower to the kidneys.

WARM FEBRILE DISEASES Wen Bing 温病 Generally refers to diseases brought about by pathogenic external heat factors. Features are acute onset, marked fever and heat symptoms, drastic changes, and significant impact on the yin aspects of the body, i.e. body fluids etc.

YANG EXHAUSTION Wang Yang 亡阳 A critical condition in which there is depletion of yang Qi. The clinical pattern manifests itself as profuse sweating, aversion to cold, cold extremities, a pale facial complexion, shortness of breath and a superficial, weak and rapid pulse.

YANG QI 阳气 The counterpart of yin Qi. It is a manifestation of external hyperactivity, light, ascending, clearing, strengthening Qi.

YIN QI 阴气 The opposite of yang Qi. It is a manifestation of internal, descending, inhibiting, undermining, turbid Qi.

VITAL FLUIDS or BODY FLUIDS Jin ye 津液 This refers to all the fluid constituents of the body.

BIBLIOGRAPHY

CHAPTER I: THE PRACTICE OF TRADITIONAL CHINESE MEDICINE

Cheng, Y.R. (1983), *An Interpretation of the Treatise on Febrile Diseases*, 伤寒论阐释, Shanxi Science and Technology Publishing House, Shanxi, China

Compilation Committee of the New Edition of Dictionary On Philosophy (1991), *New Edition of Dictionary On Philosophy*, 新编哲学大辞典, Harbin Publishing House, Harbin, China

Compiling Group (1971), *New China Chinese Character Dictionary*, 新华字典, Commercial Press Beijing, China

Deng, T.T. (1987), *TCM Diagnostic Discipline*, 中医诊断学, People's Medicine Publishing House, Beijing, China

Deng, W.J. (1988), *On the Clinical Patterns of Pain*, 痛证论, South China Engineering University Publishing House, Kwangzhow, China

Guo, G.C. (1991), *Dictionary on the Yellow Emperor's Inner Canons*, 黄帝内经词典, Tianjin Science and Technology Publishing House, Tianjin, China

He, Z.Q. (1991), *Modern TCM Internal Medicine Discipline*, 现代中医内科学, China TCM Science and Technology Publishing House, Beijing, China

Jia, D.D. (1979), *An Outline History of Medicine in China*, Shanxi Province People's Publishing House, Shanxi, China

Peng, G.L. (1986), *Concise Ancient Chinese Character Dictionary*, 简明古汉语字典, Sichuan People's Publishing House, Sichuan, China

TCM Research Institute (1985), *TCM Diagnostic Discipline of Differentiating Symptoms and Signs*, 中医症状鉴别诊断学 People's Medicine Publishing House, Beijing, China

Tiquia, R. (1994), 'Developing Criteria For TCM Standards in Australia', *Pacific Journal of Oriental Medicine* (2), p. 38–45

Turnbull, D. (1993), 'The Ad-hoc Collective Work of Building Gothic Cathedrals with Templates, Strings & Geometry'; *Science Technology and Human Values* (18), 3, pp. 322–24

Weiger, L. (1965), *Chinese Characters*, Paragon Book Reprint Group, New York p. 224

Wu, J.R. (1979), *A Chinese-English Dictionary*, Commercial Press, Beijing, China

Zhao, E.J. (1987), *TCM Discipline on Clinical Pattern Diagnosis and Treatment*, 中医证候诊断治疗学, Tianjin Science and Technology Publishing House, Tianjin, China

Zhao, F. (1981), *Detailed Exposition On the Fundamental Theories of TCM*, 中医基础理论详解, Fujian Science and Technology Publishing House, Fujian, China

CHAPTER II: A BRIEF HISTORY OF TCM

Cheng, S.D. (1982), *Annotated Compilations of the Plain Questions, Canons of Medicine*, 素问注释汇悴, People's Medicine Publishing House, Beijing, China

Chimin, K.W. (1936), *The History of Chinese Medicine*, National Quarantine Service, Shanghai, China

English Dept of the Beijing Medical Academy (1979), *A Chinese-English Dictionary of Commonly Used Medical Terminology*, 汉英常用医学词汇, People's Medicine Publishing House, Beijing, China

Fu, W.K. (1985), *Traditional Chinese Medicine and Pharmacology*, Foreign Languages Press, Beijing, China

Fu, W.K. (1988), *The Story of Chinese Acupuncture and Moxibustion*, Foreign Languages Press, Beijing, China

Guo, G.C. (1991), *Yellow Emperor's Canons On Medicine Dictionary*, 黄帝内经词典, Tianjin Science and Technology Publishing House, Tianjin, China

Hebei Province Medical Institute (1984), *Canons on Acupuncture-Annotated (Vols I and II)*, 灵枢经校释, People's Medicine Publishing House, Beijing, China

Institute of the History of Natural Sciences, Chinese Academy of Sciences (1983), *Ancient China's Technology and Science*, Foreign Languages Press, Beijing, China

Jia, D.D. (1979), *A Brief History of Chinese Medicine*, 中国医学史略, Shanxi People's Publishing House, Shanxi, China

Jian, B. (1964), *A Concise History of China*, Foreign Languages Press, Beijing, China

Kaptchuck, T.J. (1983), *The Web That Has No Weaver*, Gordon and Weed, New York

Li, J.W. (1989), *A Brief History of Ancient Chinese Medicine*, 中国古代医学史略, Hebei Province Science and Technology Publishing House, Hebei, China

Liu, H.T. (1991), *History of Ancient Chinese Science and Technology*, 中国古代科技史, Nankai University Publishing House, Tianjin, China

Liu, N.C. (1983), *General Principles in TCM Dialectics*, 中医学辨证法概论, Guangdong Provincial Science and Technology Publication, Guangdong, China

Liu, N.S. (1991), 'The Artistic Charm of the Chinese Character' in *Papers on Conference On The Chinese Language and Chinese Character*, Vol I, Jilin Education Publishig House, Jilin, China

Meng, J.C. (1991), *Introduction to TCM*, 中医学概论, People's Medicine Publishing House, Beijing, China, p. 9–10

Ou, M. (1988), *Chinese-English Dictionary of Traditional Chinese Medicine*, Joint Publishing (HK) Co Ltd, Hong Kong

Ronan, C.A. (1978), *The Shorter Science and Civilization in China: An Abridgement of Joseph Needham's Original Text*, Cambridge University Press, Cambridge

Si, Y.Y. (1984), *History of Medicine in China*, 中国医学史, People's Medicine Publishing House, Beijing, China

Tang, K.J., (1992), *Ancient Chinese Language,* 古代汉语, Beijing Publishing House, Beijing, China

Wieger, L. (1965), *Chinese Characters,* Paragon Book Reprint Corp, New York

Wu, J.R. (1979), *A Chinese-English Dictionary,* 汉英词典, Commercial Press, Beijing, China

Yan, S., Zhang, S.C. (1985), *Records of TCM and Western Medicine In Combination,* Vol II, 医学衷中参西绿, Hebei Province Science and Technology Publication, Hebei, China

Zhao, Y.J. (1984), *TCM Clinical Patterns Diagnosis and Therapeutics,* 中医证候诊断治疗学, Tianjin Science and Technology Publishing House, Tianjin, China

Zhen, Z.Y. (1984), *History of Chinese Medicine,* 中国医学史, Shanghai Science and Technology Publishing House, Shanghai, China

Zhou, Y.M. (1983), *Famous Doctors of Various Historical Eras Discuss Medical Ethics,* 历代名医论医德, Hunan Province Science and Technology Publishing House, Hunan, China

CHAPTER III: TCM OUTSIDE CHINA

Ackerknecht E.H. (1982), *A Short History of Medicine,* John Hopkins University Press, Baltimore

Acupuncture Ethics and Standards Organisation, *Codes of Ethics and Standards of Practice*

Farquhar, J. (1987), 'Problems of Knowledge In Contemporary Chinese Medical Discourse', in *Social Science and Medicine* (24) 12, pp.1013–1021

Loh, M. (1985), 'Victoria As Catalyst For Western and Chinese Medicine', in *Journal of Royal Historical Society of Victoria,* pp. 40-41

CHAPTER IV: CHINESE HERBAL MEDICINE

Beijing College of TCM (1980), *The Chemical Components of Chinese Herbs,* 中草药成分化学, People's Health Publishing House, Beijing, China

Bensky, D. (1986), *Chinese Herbal Medicine, Materia Medica,* Eastland Press, Seattle, pp. vii-ix

Bi, Y. (1984), *Historical Materials On Chinese Herbal Medicine,* 中国药学史料, People's Health Publishing House, Beijing, China

Bo, Y.D. (1984), *Elaboration of Chinese Herbal Prescriptions,* 医方发挥, Liaoning Province Scientific and Technical Publishing House, Liaoning Province, China

Dou, G.X. (1987), *Your TCM Adviser,* 您的中医顾问, Jiangsu Provincial Scientific and Technical Publishing House, Jiangsu Province, China

Guo, S.Z. (1992), *Dictionary of Toxic Herbs,* 有毒中草药大辞典, Tianjin City Science and Technological Translation and Publishing Company, Tianjin, China

Liang, Y.W. (1975), *Application of Concepts of Combining Chinese Herbs,* 中药配伍应用, Inner Mongolian People's Publishing House, Inner Mongolia, China

Liu, F. (1980), *Chinese Medical Terminology*, The Commercial Press Ltd., Kowloon, Hong Kong

Liu, S.S. (1975), *Excerpts of Research Literature On Chinese Herbs*, 1820–1961, 中药研究文献摘要, Scientific Publication, Beijing, China

National Intermediate Health Schools Experimental Teaching Materials Compiling Group For Chinese Herbal Medicine (1979), *Chinese Herbal Medicine*, 中草药学, Guangdong People's Publishing House, Guangdong, China

Si, Y.Y. (1984), *History of Chinese Medicine*, 中国医学史, People's Health Publishing House, Beijing, China

Tau, D.P. (1990), 'Literary Review of 54 Articles On Adverse Reaction From Chinese Herbs', *China Medicinal Herb Journal* (15) 4, pp. 53–56

Tao, N.G. (1985), *A Required Reading On Herb Decoction And Administration*, 煎服中药必读, Shandong Provincial Scientific and Technical Publishing House, Shandong, China

The TCM Herb Prescription Compiling Group of Sun Yat Sen Medical School (1981), *Selected Lectures in Chinese Herb Prescriptions*, 中医方剂选讲, Guangdong Provincial Scientific and Technical Publishing House, Guangdong Province, China

Tiquia, R. (1985), 'Chinese Medicinal Herbs', in *Australian Wellbeing* (6) Jan–Feb., pp. 31–34

Yan, Z.H. (1984), *Chinese Herbal Medicine For Clinical Use*, 临床实用中药学, People's Health Publishing House, Beijing, China

Yan, Z.H. (1991), *Chinese Herbal Medicine*, 中医学, People's Health Publishing House, Beijing, China

Yao, J.N. (1984), *Preparation and Processing of Raw Chinese Herbs*, 中药的炮制, Kwangdong Science and Technology Publishing House, Kwangdong, China

Zhao, F. (1981), *Detailed Exposition Of the Fundamental Theories of TCM*, 中医基础理论详解, Fujian Scientific and Technical Publishing House, Fujian Province, China

Zhu, J.H. (1991), *Mutual Interactions Between Chinese Natural Substances and Western Pharmaceutical Drugs*, 中西药物相互作用, People's Medicine Publishing House, Beijing, p. 49

Zhu, Y.F. (1991), *A Handbook On Detoxification Of Chinese Medicinal Herbs and Herbal Preparations*, 中药中成药解毒手册, People's Army Medicine Publishing House, Beijing, China

CHAPTER V: FOOD THERAPY

Cai, J.F. (1988), *Eating Your Way To Health*, Foreign Languages Press, Beijing, China

Dou, G.X. (1979), *A Compass On Food Therapy*, 饮食治疗指南, Jiangsu Province Science and Technology Publishing House, Jiangsu, China

Hu, S.H. (1330), annot. and trans. into modern Mandarin by C.F. Li (1988), *Essentials of Eating and Diet*, 饮膳正要, China Commercial Press Publishing House, Beijing, China

Huang, D.S. (1987), *Recipes On Health Tonifying Medicinal Foods and Herbs*, 滋补中药保健菜谱, Science and Technology Literary Publishing House (Chongqing Branch), Chongqing, China

Jiang, Z. (1985), *Practical TCM Study on Nutrition*, 实用中医营养学, People's Liberation Army Publishing House, Beijing, China

Li, Z.G. (1991), *Recipes For Nurturing Life for Everyone*, 大众养生食谱, Light Industry Publishing House, Beijing, China

Lu, H.C. (1986), *Chinese System of Food Cures*, Sterling Publishing Co., New York

Pang, M.Q. (1986), *Almanac On Chinese Herb and Food Recipes*, 中国药膳大全, Sichuan Province Science and Technology Publishing House, Sichuan, China

Peng, M.Q. (1984), *Medicinal Food for Everyone*, 大众药膳, Sichuan Science and Technology Publishing House, Sichuan, China

Qian, B.W. (1987), *Chinese Study On Food Therapy*, 中国食疗学, Shanghai Science and Technology Publishing House, Shanghai, China

Rinzler, C. (1987), *Food Facts*, Bloomsbury, London

Sun, B.Q. (1979), *Common Foods Used for Medicinal Purposes*, 常见药用食物, Shanxi Province Publishing House, Shanxi, China

Tiquia, R. (Nov./Dec.1985), 'Food Therapy', *Australian Wellbeing* (11), pp. 32–36

Tiquia, R. (27 Oct.1987), 'The Chinese Way to Restore The Body's Harmony', *The Age*, p. 41

Weng, W.J. *Food Tonification and Food Therapy*, 食补与食疗, Popular Science Publishing House, Beijing, China

Zhang, J.J. (1981), *Food And Curing Diseases*, 食物与治病, Popular Science Publishing House (Guangzhou branch) Guangzhou, China

Zhang, Z.L. (1984), *Vegetables for Medicinal Use*, 药用蔬菜, Guangxi Provincial People's Publishing House, Guangxi, China

CHAPTER VI: THE PRACTICE OF ACUPUNCTURE

Dou, G.X. (1985), *Your TCM Adviser*, 您的中医顾问, Jiangsu Province Science and Technology Publishing House, Jiangsu, China

Fu, Q. (1991), *Complete Works On Practical Acupuncture and Moxibustion Clinical Therapy*, 实用针久疗法临床大全, China TCM and Pharmacology Publishing House, Beijing, China

Fu, W.K. (1975), *The Story of Chinese Acupuncture and Moxibustion*, Foreign Languages Press, Beijing, China

Hebei Province Medical College (1984), *Annotated Spiritual Axis* (Vols I and II), 灵枢经校释, People's Medical Publishing House, Beijing, China

Jiao, G.R. (1981), *Summary of Acupuncture and Moxibustion Clinical Experience*, 针灸临床经验辑要, People's Medical Publishing House, Beijing, China

Li, S.Z. (1983), *Clinical Elaboration of Common Acupuncture Points*, 常用俞穴临床发挥, People's Medical Publishing House, Beijing, China

Liu, H.Y., (1988), *Complete Work On Practical Acupuncture*, 实用针灸大全, Beijing Publishing House, Beijing, China

Lu, S.K. *One Hundred Manipulation Techniques in Acupuncture*, 针刺手法一百种, China Medical Scientific and Technological Publishing House, Beijing, China

Meng, Z.W. (1983), 'The Acupuncture Channels — the Network of The Third Equilibrium', 第三平衡系统 — 经络系统, *Chinese Acupuncture and Moxibustion* (3) 1, p. 25–26

Regional Working Group On the Standardization of Acupuncture Nomenclature (1984), *Standard Acupuncture Nomenclature*, WHO Regional Office For Western Pacific, Manila, Philippines

Shanghai College of Traditional Chinese Medicine, trans. J. O'Connor, et al. (1981), *Acupuncture a Comprehensive Text*, Eastland Press, Chicago

Shen, D.K. (1989), 'Research on the Morphological Structure Involved in Acupuncture Sensation', *Acta Medica Sinica*, 中国中医药学报 (4) 4, pp 57–64

Shi, Z.X. (1984), 'Seriously Prevent Acupuncture-Related Accidents and Complications', 严防针刺意外损伤辑并发证, *Chinese Acupuncture and Moxibustion* (284) 6, pp. 40–41

TCM Research Academy (1981), *Progress in Acupuncture Research*, 中国研究进展, People's Medical Publishing House, Beijing, China

Tiquia, R. (29 Aug. 1988), 'Sounds From Within', *The Age*

Tiquia, R. (19 Dec. 1988), 'Missing The Point On Acupuncture', *The Age*

Tiquia, R. (17 Sept. 1990), 'Studies Reveal Point of Acupuncture', *The Australian*, p. 8

Wang, X.T. (1988), *Complete Works of Chinese Acupuncture and Moxibustion*, Vol I, 中国针灸大全, Henan Province Science and Technology Publishing House, Henan, China

Wieger, L. (1965), *Chinese Characters*, Paragon Book Reprint Corp., New York

Yang, J.Z. (1601), Heilongjiang Province Motherland Medical Research Institute (annot. 1984), *Compendium of Acupuncture and Moxibustion*, 针灸大全, People's Medical Publishing House, Beijing, China

CHAPTER VII: TUINA: CHINESE THERAPEUTIC MASSAGE

Anhui Medical School, trans. M.L Hor et al. (1983), *Chinese Massage Therapy*, Second Back Row Press, Australia

Ji, G.J. (1981), *Tuina — A Simplified Compilation*, 推拿简编, People's Medical Publishing House, Beijing, China

Li, S.Z. (1983), *Clinical Elaboration of Common Acupuncture Points*, 常用俞穴临床发挥, People's Medical Publishing House, Beijing, China

Li, Y.C. (1985), *The Art of Chinese Massage*, 中国按摩术, Anhui Province Science and Technology Publishing House, Anhui, China

Luo, J.H. (1987), *Chinese Tuina Medicine History — Origins of Manipulation Techniques*, 中华推拿医学志—手法源流, Science and Technological Literature Publishing House (Chongqing Branch), Chongqing, China

Luo, J.H. (1990), *A Hundred Methods of Practical Tuina In Treating Diseases*, 实用推拿治病百法, People's Sport Publishing House, Beijing, China

Sports Medicine Dept. of the Hospital Attached To The Anhui Medical College (1982), *Tuina Therapy and Therapeutic Exercise Training*, 推拿疗法与医疗练功, People's Medical Publishing House, Beijing, China

Tiquia, R. (1986), *Chinese Infant Massage*, Greenhouse Publication, Melbourne

Wang, Y.R. (1985), *Family Massage To Treat Disease and For Health*, 家庭按摩治病与健康, Knowledge Publishing House, Beijing, China

Yu, D.F. (1985), *TCM Discipline of Tuina*, 中医推拿学, People's Medical Publishing House, Beijing, China

Zhang, Y.Y. (1991), *Almanac On Chinese Massage*, 中国按摩大全, Tianjin University Publishing House, Tianjin, China

CHAPTER VIII: NURTURING LIFE

Cao, X.L. (1981), *The Chinese Art of Physical Building*, 中国健身术, Shanxi Province Science and Technology Publishing House, Shanxi, China

China Reconstructs Press (1989), *Practical Ways to Good Health Through Chinese Traditional Medicine*, China Reconstructs Press, Beijing, China

Dai, X.M. (1986), *Wishing You Health and Longevity*, 祝您健康长寿, Nankai University Publishing House, Nankai, China

Dou, G.X. (1985), *Your TCM Adviser*, Jiangsu Province Science and Technology Publishing House, Jiangsu, China

Hu, B. (1982), *A Brief Introduction to the Science of Breathing Exercises*, Hai Feng Publishing Company, Hong Kong

Jiang, H.Q. (1986), *Hua Tuo's Five Animal Exercises*, 华佗五禽戏, Liaoning Province Science and Technology Publishing House, Shenyang City, China

Jolan, C. (1977), *The Tao of Love and Sex*, Dutton Paperback, New York

Liu, Z.W. (1989), *Chinese Discipline of Nurturing Life*, 中国养生学, Shanghai TCM College Publishing House, Shanghai, China

Luo, S.M. *Historical Statements On the Ancient Art of Nurturing Life and Longevity*, 古代养生长寿史话, Huang Shan Book Shop Publishing House, Hefei City, China

People's Medical Publishing House (1984), *The Chinese Way to A Long and Healthy Life*, Joint Publishing Co., Hong Kong

Tiquia, R. (1985), 'Living in Harmony', *Australian Wellbeing* (9), pp. 80–85

Tiquia, R. (1986), 'Qi – The Energy of Life', *Australian Wellbeing* (16), pp. 102–106

Tiquia, R. (27 Oct. 1987), 'Chinese Way to Restore the Body's Harmony', *The Age*, p. 41

Wang, L. (1988), *Essential Key To Ancient and Contemporary Man-Woman Art of Nurturing Life*, 古今男女养生精要, International Culture Publishing Company, Beijing, China

Wei, D.X. (1984), *A Chapter On The Tao of Longevity*, 寿道篇, Henan Province Science and Technology Publishing House, Henan, China

Zhang, M.W. (1985), *The Chinese Qigong Therapy*, Shandong Science and Technology Press, Jinan, China

Zhao, F. (1981), *Detailed Exposition On the Fundamental Theories of TCM*, 中医基础理论详解, Fujian Science and Technology Publishing House, Fujian, China

GLOSSARY OF TERMS

Beijing Medical College (1984), *Dictionary of Traditional Chinese Medicine*, The Commercial Press Ltd, Hong Kong

Deng, T.Z. (1987), *TCM Discipline On Diagnosis*, 中医诊断学, People's Medicine Publishing House, Beijing, China

English Language Faculty of the Beijing Medical College (1982), *Chinese-English Dictionary on Commonly Used Medical Terminology*, 汉英常用医学词汇, People's Medicine Publishing House, Beijing, China

Ou, M. (1988), *Chinese-English Dictionary of Traditional Chinese Medicine*, Joint Publishing (HK) Co. Ltd, Hong Kong

TCM Dictionary Compiling Group (1986), *Concise TCM Dictionary*, 简明中医辞典, People's Medicine Publishing House, Beijing, China

INDEX